Toughen Up

Zero fuss fitness

Ian Oliver

snowbooks

Proudly published in 2009 by

Snowbooks Ltd., 120 Pentonville Road, London, N1 9JN

email: info@snowbooks.com

www.snowbooks.com

British Library Cataloguing in Publication Data

A catalogue record for this book is available from the British Library.

ISBN 9781906727130

Printed and bound in China through Worldprint.

By the same author

ISBN 9781905005314   ISBN 9780954575984   ISBN 9781905005161

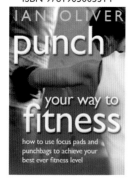 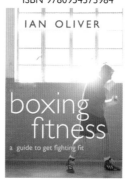 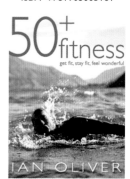

(all available from Snowbooks)

Contents

Foreword

Working (if you could call it work) at The Bob Breen Academy as strength, conditioning and boxing coach, my main function is to get people from all walks of life in shape to participate in Mixed Martial Arts or Boxing. One indisputable fact that most of my students must face is that they will need to "toughen up". It is very often the prime reason they first arrive at the gym.

I hope the fitness advice in this book, which is comprised of various aspects of the training I advise my students to adopt, can take the reader on the same path to the level of strength and conditioning that gives the self-confidence and the assurance to face the slings and arrows of modern living.

Ian Oliver

May 2009

I shall be telling this with a sigh
Somewhere ages and ages hence;
Two roads diverged in a wood, and I –
I took the one less travelled by,
And that has made the difference.

Robert Frost (1874-1963) *The Road Not Taken*.

Dedication

Dedicated to all instructors, staff and students of the Bob Breen Academy, past and present.

To Brenda, Marge, Sue, Jimmy, Tom, Glen, Becky, Ellie, Joe, Clare, Danny, Ronnie, Ruby, The Mitchells and The Walkers.

To the memory of John McDavid, Laura Logan, Andrew "Wink" Walker, Roy Beckworth, Johnny Bird, Johnny Hill, John Davis, Jack Sheriff, Mag and Archie, Dolly and Ernie, F.S.O. and Roger Barnes.

Acknowledgements

Pete Drinkell (yet again) for his terrific photography

Emma at Snowbooks, for just about everything

Bob and Judy for use of The Academy

All my Monday students at The Academy

Terry Barnett, Wayne Rowlands, Owen Ogbourne, Dave Birkett, Bob Breen, Savash Mustafa and Steve "Mr Kettlebells" Wright for help and advice.

All the instructors and students of the Academy who graciously gave of their time to model for photographs.

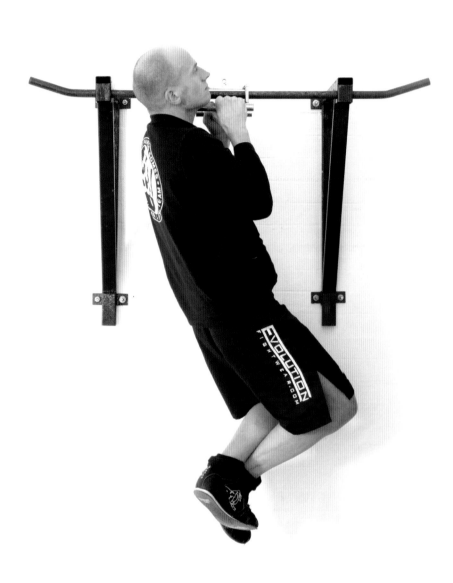

Introduction

Notes

- Age is no barrier to achieving fitness, as long as you are healthy.

- Cost is no barrier as throughout this book I endeavour to provide affordable alternatives to gym membership, although I consider gym membership to be money well invested – your health should be a principal investment. Merely having a gym membership will not get you fit – you actually need to turn up there and train regularly.

- Training will be easier if you have a history of sports/fitness, otherwise you may have to be prepared for the long haul – but it can be achieved.

- It is advisable to get clearance from your doctor if you have any doubts about your medical condition or your medication prior to training.

- It is even more advisable, in fact paramount, for anybody who does not intend to do any exercise to obtain a doctor's clearance!

How bad do you want it?

If you have decided it is time to "toughen up" you must bear in mind that it will involve hard work, sacrifice and some unpleasant choices, especially regarding diet for many participants. You will have to become acquainted with solid, hardworking – even punishing – routines; takeaways should become a virtual stranger.

In this book I have tried to impart the information I use in the gym where I have trained clients and friends for many years. If you are expecting significant amounts of technical and biological data to substantiate my advice I fear you have come to the wrong publication: I try to keep things as simple as possible, and stick to that which I have found actually works. I have found that to get results you have to work for it. Nice, easy exercise will not bring about positive progression.

If you pick up a glossy magazine that promises to get you a "beach body" in six weeks, ask yourself "is this very likely to happen for me?" The answer is that if you spent six weeks doing day-long hard labour fed only on a fat-free diet it might be a possibility. The reality is that it is going to take months, and progress will be dictated by the acronym "F.I.T.T.":

F = frequency (how often you train)
I = intensity (how much effort you put in)
T = time (how much time you spend training)
T = type of training (which parts of the body it works)

An important point to remember is that rest is just as important as training. You will need time to recuperate from the work you put in; failure to do so only results in muscle soreness and eventually disappointment, since the soreness makes training impossible.

Try to plan your training to fit in with your life-style, but be prepared to make your lifestyle fit in with your training if you are serious about getting a satisfactory outcome. Which brings me back to the original question, "How bad do you want it?" Maybe this is where you will find out.

My (much) younger colleagues jest that I have been doing this stuff for such a long time that my early training programmes were in Latin, and I have to admit it does seem like eons, but that time has given me a chance to watch people I often despaired of ever getting fit finally becoming stronger, faster, healthier and more self-confident than I had ever given them credit for, which has been heartening. I hope I can do the same for you.

Your possible reasons for 'taking the hard(er) road'

» 'I used to be fit and healthy but if I'm honest I have to admit in recent times I've turned into something of a slob.'

» 'I've never been fit or healthy, have always avoided exercise like the plague, but have tired of being regarded, even by myself, as a slob.'

» 'I've run out of excuses such as "I'm big-boned", "it's my glands", "I'm genetically cursed with being overweight", and realise it's *me*, and I have to take some direct action.'

» 'I want to have the odd social drink/glass of wine occasionally without feeling like an arch criminal.'

» 'My partner has been making less than subtle hints about improving my size/condition.'

» 'My holiday/leisure wear consists mainly of dark tops and baggy shorts in an attempt to minimise my "overflows." I've taken to wearing black in an attempt to minimise my lumpy appearance.'

» 'My father and his father both died of heart failure before they were 60. I intend to have a strong heart when I reach that age as my best form of life insurance.'

» 'I've given up smoking, cut back drastically on booze and need to kick-start a new routine to start showing some positive improvement by setting myself new goals.'

The last reason gives an insight into what is going to be required to keep you on track: a goal. You should have a target of some kind to aim at, be it fitness, weight loss (nowhere near as important as fitness) or improvement in sporting ability.

Aim at realistic targets – halving your weight, or becoming a professional boxer/footballer, are more likely to be dreams, so choose something attainable.

Pick sensible targets for weight loss, strength gain, stamina improvement and so on as opposed to the unattainable, which will only lead to disappointment, loss of self confidence and, ultimately, failure.

If personal problems are mounting up or times are just proving difficult it always seems that these setbacks can best be faced if you can get yourself in the kind of shape that will reinforce your self-confidence and regain your personal pride. Many people have, in my experience, found that conditioning, and the resultant sense of well-being, go a long way to sorting your life out.

Reasons people find not to train

1. Time

'I have a hectic lifestyle, family commitments etc. When I'm not working, I really couldn't fit anything else in.'

Time management is crucial. Training needs to be structured to fit your lifestyle, but it will inevitably require some amount of sacrifice. It may be a case of giving up a large amount of the leisure time you afford yourself, possibly including the TV, cinema, football or other sports events. Try to put it into perspective and decide where your priorities lie; if you can talk yourself out of training by saying "I would if I could, but I can't find time," you will always use this as a cop-out. Getting into serious shape takes both time and effort and, if you have the willpower, you will find a way to shoehorn in the time. It may mean getting up earlier or going to bed later to cram more time into your day but that hour[*] each day could make a massive difference to your well-being and appearance. If you allocate the time, I will be able to show you how to use it to maximum effect.

2. Cost

'I can't afford to pay gym fees or buy a lot of training kit.'

---

[*]   allowing time for a quick shower/change.

If you really can't afford gym fees then you have two ways to go:

» Cut out something else. At the time of writing the average gym fee is between £25 – £60 a month. Some gyms will actually barter with you, especially if you go in a group; rather than lose 3-4 members they will sometimes offer a 'group rate'. I speak from experience and feel it's worth considering if you have some like-minded friends thinking of joining a gym.

If, however, you are going to the gym on your own, or the gym has an inflexible pricing policy – something else will have to go. A £30 a month gym is going to set you back £7.50 a week; balance that against a round of drinks, a restaurant meal, a takeaway, a club or cinema visit and consider which is the best investment for your money.

» Train at home. As long as you have room for weights (as well as a substantial floor), an exercise ball or similar kit, training at home can bring positive results. Second hand weights equipment works just as well as new gear and local papers are usually crammed with them. Running and exercising in a public park is much more beneficial than any air-conditioned gym, as long as the weather is reasonably clement. I don't advocate that anybody trains in a thunderstorm or blizzard – it comes down to common sense. Jogging/running and cycling in the park is free, and swimming at a local baths is usually inexpensive.

As for training kit, you need only shoes (running shoes are fine for gym use as well as just running), t-shirts (budget ones work fine for training – they are only going to get sweaty anyway), track bottoms/shorts according to weather conditions or personal preference.

3. Enjoyment factor

'I hate exercise, I get bored quickly.'

To get results, some degree of sacrifice needs to be made but this does not mean you have, necessarily, to be bored out of your wits or begin to lose the will to live. Try new forms of exercise or, if indoors, put some upbeat invigorating music on the stereo; at the gym put your iPod/mp3 player on and switch to something you enjoy listening to and that is likely to lift your mood. Try exercise classes you wouldn't normally consider: you might just enjoy yourself. Most men consider these classes too "girly", but look around the average gym and note that not only do the women outnumber the men, but they are, in general, in better shape. The worst you can do is hold your hands up after 10 minutes or so, admit it is not for you, make your apologies and leave quietly, telling yourself "at least I tried".

If you feel you will become bored just following one particular exercise I would suggest trying cross-training, where you can switch exercises. It's intended primarily to prevent strains, but it is also good for relieving tedium.

4. Awkwardness factor

'I've never been to the gym and wouldn't know where to start.'

You start by going to the gym and telling them exactly that: i.e. "I don't know where to start". Remember that even the most competent and confident-looking gym members had to start somewhere – they weren't born and raised there, even if some of them give that appearance. The gym should then allocate you a trainer to get you started with a simple training plan that you will be guided through; if they know you are a complete novice they will know just how to pitch the level of exercise you can cope with. A good gym will usually give you a fitness test and need to know your medical history before allowing you to commence training. They should also try to establish just why you have come to the gym; what your aims and desires are in taking the first step. I always ask people "why are you here?" It is amazing that so many individuals have so many differing reasons – "my wife complains I've got too heavy and as a result I snore loudly", "I'm/my daughter is getting married and I want to look the part on the day", or quite commonly "my doctor advised me to get some exercise". Examining your reasons for training makes sense not only for you, but for gym member retention. A fitness test is essential; having somebody keel over in front of other members is not exactly healthy for business.

5. Injury factor

'I've got a chronic injury to my back/knee/shoulder etc.'

A good trainer will find an exercise for you that will not aggravate your problem but still manage to elevate your fitness level e.g. getting you training on an exercise bike or a rowing machine. In the meantime, if you haven't had much joy from your local health practice then try seeing an osteopath or chiropractor and let them take a look at your injury. They may also be able to recommend suitable exercise for you. To put it bluntly – you need to exercise the parts that don't hurt. Even limited exercise is better than none at all.

Conclusion

Anybody can train, barring medical advice or severe lack of mobility. All you need is a good reason – health, image or otherwise – and a desire to prove to yourself, and nobody else, that you can do it.

How do I know this?

I've made it my business as a fitness professional (back when we were called gym instructors) over the last God-knows-how-long to find out what people want – not what I think they want – and then do everything in my power to help them achieve it. Some do and some do not – it all comes down to the individual's adherence to the task in hand. Personally speaking, I loved training, be it football, boxing or martial arts, and never knowingly dodged a session, even if it meant missing a big match/ fight on TV. This led my close family and friends to consider me borderline certifiably insane, possibly with some justification – and many still feel this way. Be careful – training can become addictive, but I am of the opinion it's about the best addiction there is.

Getting started

IF YOU'VE GOT THIS FAR THEN I AM going to assume you are on board for some serious, structured exercise that is going to make a drastic difference to your health, image and state of well-being, not to mention your feelings of self-confidence and self-worth.

When you decide to get involved in fitness, there are three basic areas to consider for a balanced overall improvement:

> » Cardiovascular fitness – running, swimming, cycling etc.

> » Resistance – weight training, body weight exercises (such as press-ups), most 'core' exercises.

> » Flexibility – stretching and joint mobilisation.

To the above I would add a set of exercises I like to describe as "dynamic power", for which I have included elements of Plyometric Training and Boxing Fitness. These not only add a variation to regular weight lifting, running, and so on, but to many people will offer a fresh attitude to working out, one they may never have encountered before, and will hopefully find innovative and refreshing.

I also have added Circuit Training, something I have always taught and swear by, for one basic reason – I know it works. I have seen the results over a good many years. It is a variation on training aimed at working all areas and aspects of fitness.

Sports & Fitness

Regular training in the sport of your choice may possibly get you strong and fit, but only if the effort you put in is going to make you sweat and exercise your heart, lungs and major muscle groups. You can thus rule out the obvious, such as darts and snooker, but at the same time golf and tennis doubles (though I love them both) are not going to make a significant difference. People tend to be wary of such sports as squash as they have all heard of somebody going face down with a heart attack on the court, but, like running fatalities and footballers who have dropped dead, it is not the sport that killed them, but coronary heart disease. To play squash you need to be in good shape. The same applies to any vigorous sport and to long-distance running. It is therefore essential that anybody considering taking up a physically demanding sport takes stock of their personal fitness. While running the London Marathon some years back I was astonished at the large number of people who were reduced to walking after just a few miles. Clearly they had not trained specifically for this event and had given very little thought to just how hard it would be to compete efficiently.

Vigorous sports can help get you in shape, but first be certain you are already in good enough shape to take part in them. Always err on the side of caution. You have the rest of your life to get fit (you will hear this again).

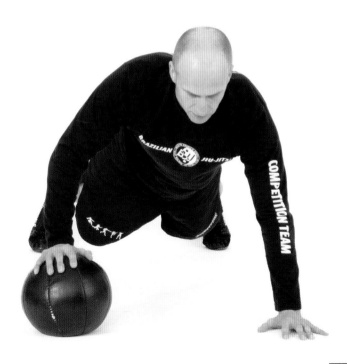

Fitness self-testing

IT IS A GOOD IDEA TO ESTABLISH HOW fit or unfit you are at the out-set of a training regime. It means you can chart your progress, and as I realise you are unlikely to want to fiddle about with dreary calculations, I have made it very simple.

The example below shows the first three weekly tests of an actual subject (name has been changed to protect the innocent). This was the result of him training on light weights, moderate cardiovascular work and one boxing workout per week.

In order to keep your own records, some tests require basic equipment, listed below.

This equipment is hardly up to N.A.S.A standard, but it will be fine for your purposes.

SAMPLE SELF-TEST. SEE END OF BOOK FOR PHOTOCOPIABLE BLANK VERSION.

	FITNESS TEST	1	2	3
1	BLOOD PRESSURE	133/78	136/86	130/83
2	PULSE	68	66	62
3	PEAK FLOW	700	710	715
4	BODY FAT	30.9	30.5	28.75
5	WEIGHT	15st	14st 8lb	14st 5lb
6	WAIST	44	41	39
7	HIPS	45	42	41
8	ONE MILE RUN	10.3	10.15	10.1
9	CHINS	5	7	8
10	PRESS-UPS	10	25	28
11	CURL-UPS	30	42	44
12	PLANK/BRIDGE TIME	55 seconds	57	60
13	B M I	28.5	27.5	27.5

Test

Blood Pressure. You will need a very basic blood pressure monitor. Argos have several, starting at about £15. This model will be adequate.

Pulse. You can take your own pulse by placing two fingers on your neck or wrist until you feel a beat, but if you are using a blood pressure monitor this will give you your pulse as well. Try to always take your blood pressure and pulse at the same time of day for greater accuracy, and never immediately after exercising.

Peak Flow. Check the state of your lungs by blowing into one of these meters, a familiar instrument to anybody unfortunate enough to suffer from asthma. You can pay as little as £10 for one on the web (for instance, I found one for £15 from Amazon).

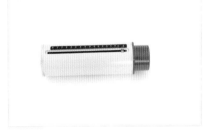

Body fat. I prefer body calipers which cost about £10, although some consider them to be a bit fiddly. The hand-held Omron Body Fat Monitor is reasonably user-friendly and costs £32-35 from Amazon.co.uk.

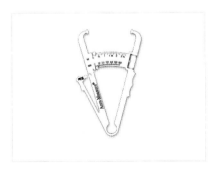

Weight. Always use the same scales. They might not be accurate, but they should at least be consistent. Always take your weight at the same time of day; everyone is usually heavier in the evening, so cheer yourself up and have a weigh-in first thing in the morning. Only weigh yourself once a week when filling in the log – don't become weight-obsessed.

RIGHT: HAND-HELD OMRON BODY FAT MONITOR

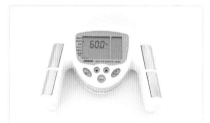

Waist & Hips. Obviously all you need is a tape measure. Take the waist measurement at navel level and hips at the widest part.

One Mile Run. You only need a watch, preferably digital, unless you are a stickler for accuracy, which will require one with a stopwatch. I'm a fan of the Casio G-Shock, costing about £50 (cheaper abroad) but Casio, Timex and Lorus all produce watches good enough for training for £20 or less. If you have a Heart Rate Monitor watch, simply use that.

Chins. If you can find a chinning bar at the gym (most have them) all well and good, but failing that Argos sell one for home use for about £8. Ensure your doorframe is strong enough to take your exertions. Count how many times you can perform a straight arm pull-up. If using the home version, you will need to start with bent knees if you are on the tall side.

BELOW: CHINNING BAR

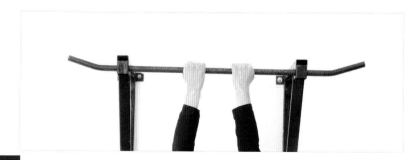

Press-ups. You just have to beat your previous personal best with each session.

Curl-ups. Again, beat your personal best. See page 88 for technique.

Plank/Bridge. Place a stopwatch within sight, rest on elbows and toes, contract your abdominals, but don't hold your breath. Beat your last effort. See page 93.

BMI. Check your BMI on http://www.nhsdirect.nhs.uk/magazine/interactive/bmi/index.aspx (or http://tinyurl.com/24a88e) where the calculation is done for you. All you need is your height and weight.

In the comments section, keep a note of how you felt, if your run was slow due to bad weather or anything you think may influence your records.

Don't beat yourself up if the results are not outstanding at first. Just tell yourself that you have the rest of your life to get fit.

Tips:

» Take your pulse first thing in the morning before taking any tea or coffee, ideally before you actually get out of bed so it is, in reality, a "resting pulse".

» Always take your weight at the same time of day, but only once a week. Everybody actually weighs more by evening time: you'll feel much happier with an early morning weigh-in. Weighing yourself daily, wherein there is usually only minimal change, can prove dispiriting – stick to once a week.

» Take your blood pressure when you are at rest, and never just after exercise.

Keep an Exercise Record/Log

One way to continually prod yourself into activity is to keep a training diary. All you need is a pocket diary (or a desk diary if you intend to write down all your weight training exercises, reps and sets). Every time you work out, write down:

- date & time (and weather conditions if training outdoors)

- what exercise

- how you felt (including any twinges)

- record of progress

If you are trying to lose some weight then also keep a food diary alongside your exercise diary. You can work out roughly how many calories you have taken on in total by counting your intake from food and subtracting your energy expenditure.

Consider the amount of calories expended on the activities shown on the right; they will vary with your size and how much effort you apply.

Activity	Calories Minute
Driving car	2.8
Driving motor bike	3.4
Painting	3.5
Vacuuming	3.5
Sweeping floors	3.9
Ironing	4.2
Gardening (weeding)	5.6
Gardening (digging)	8.6
Cycling (easy)	5.0
Cycling (hard)	15
Dancing (leisurely)	5
Dancing (vigorously)	7.5
Golf	5
Walking (3.5 m.p.h.)	6
Power walking	8-10
Jogging (5 m.p.h.)	10-12
Running (7.5 m.p.h.)	15
Aerobics	8-10
Step aerobics	9-12
Running (10m.p.h.)	20
Playing football (according to position)	12-17
Swimming (breaststroke/backstroke)	6-12
Swimming (butterfly)	14
Swimming (crawl)	9-12
Squash	11-17
Skipping rope (leisurely)	10
Skipping rope (fast)	15
Rowing (leisurely)	5
Rowing (strenuously)	15
Badminton (recreational)	5
Badminton (competitive)	10
Table tennis (recreational)	5
Table tennis (competitive)	7.5
Lawn tennis (recreational)	7
Lawn tennis (competitive)	11
Weight training (general)	8-10

Body types

Know your type

WE ALL LOOK THE WAY WE DO THANKS to our genetic make-up and our hormones. Diet and physical activity play an obvious role in our appearance, but not, you may have noticed with some bitterness, in the same way with everybody.

As a youngster I worked with a guy named Pete Eddowes, who could eat two dinners to my one in the café, and then double up on jam roly-poly and custard to finish. He had energy to burn, was forever hungry and never added an ounce of weight to his long lean frame (which he retains to this day), a talent which many colleagues considered freakishly fortunate. What we didn't realise, and he certainly didn't at the time, was that he was an 'ectomorph', one of the three main body types, categorised as soma types.

While some people fit exactly into one of the soma types, many of us are somewhere in between.

It all started back in the 1940s when William H Sheldon introduced his theory of soma types, sometimes referred to as Sheldon types. Sheldon's three main categories were:

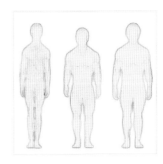

>> *Ectomorph:* usually willowy types, with narrow shoulders and hips. They are the weight-training instructors' nightmare: trying to pack muscle on to people with this frame is a real challenge, as they have a high metabolism. They usually have very low body fat levels.

» *Mesomorph:* usually densely muscled, medium to large frame, medium to high metabolism, capable of putting on muscle without too much trouble, but also fat if inactive or overfed.

» *Endomorph:* unfortunate enough to be endowed with higher body fat levels than they would like, and a problem shifting it; they have a low metabolism. They invariably have a limited amount of muscle mass and size, which usually endows them with a 'pear' shape.

However, it is not as clear-cut as all that. Most people have characteristics from the other groups in differing proportions.

The three basic groups grew into wide usage in literature involving diet, bodybuilding and general exercise, so at least some of the school sports coaches should have had some idea why some children were shaped the way they were and could not help their ample proportions. I always felt sorry for the overweight kids in gym classes; we had a P.E. master who regarded them on the same footing as war criminals, unaware of the fact that they were endomorphs doing their level best.

Conclusion

If you don't like your shape, do something about it yourself, especially if your ancestors haven't bestowed you with the appearance you would have chosen.

All is not lost. Diet and exercise can make large, if not drastic changes to your body regardless of soma type, so you can still 'shape' your own destiny. The soma types are only a guide, but they nevertheless help us to be realistic about our ambitions with regard to our figure.

Cardiovascular training

IF YOU HAVE DECIDED TO IMPROVE YOUR FITNESS then the heart and lungs are a good place to start before you worry about muscles or weight loss/gain. Cardiovascular exercise will improve your endurance and stamina – what can simply be regarded as "staying power". Running, jogging (slower running, in other words), brisk walking, swimming, cycling, skipping with a rope, dancing vigorously, aerobic classes of all sorts will make your heart beat faster and build stronger lungs, which will hopefully improve your well-being. To get stronger and fitter, however, you are going to have to work hard – really hard – at them.

I have chosen the following activities as part of your fitness regime solely because they are uncomplicated and attainable. It is pointless for me to tell you to attend classes if you live in a village miles from anywhere; unless you prefer to buy a static cycle or rowing machine, the instruction I have given here is inexpensive and achievable. In fact, I have honed it down to two cost-free disciplines (once you have lashed out a fiver on a skipping rope):

- *Running:* (progressing from jogging)

- *Skipping:* Don't dismiss this by saying "I can't skip". I have taught people to skip who appeared to have difficulty in walking and remaining upright for extended periods – trust me, it's easy! Just follow the simple instructions. It is truly beneficial. See page 54.

Alternatively:

- *Swimming:* If you have access to the swimming pool (hopefully they haven't closed yours yet to erect yet another block of tasteful apartments for inner-city living) then take full advantage of it. To achieve good results from swimming you should be moist from perspiration as well as the water from the pool.

- *Cycling:* Got a bike? Good – you'll need to think about getting some serious mileage in. A static bike is fine (there are usually a varied selection of unwanted exercise bikes listed in the "free newspaper" that is usually consigned unread to the recycling sack, so you don't have to spend a fortune on one.)

- *Rowing:* Not on the river, unless of course you can, in which case this will be excellent training. I'm thinking more on the realistic and practical lines of indoor rowing machines, such as those used in gyms, which can provide a great workout. Britain's Olympic champions, such as Messrs Redgrave and Pinsent, train on them, which should be recommendation enough.

Most common questions

How much training will I need to do to get results? How long will it take?

Taking your time

You will have to budget your time to fit in with your lifestyle; it would be facile of me to tell you to get a long run in first thing in the morning if you have to be on a building site or on duty at a hospital at seven a.m. It is, however, your responsibility to take charge of your training and set aside adequate time to fit in everything you need to do to get results, even if it means disrupting your social life. It is the easiest thing in the world to talk yourself out of training by blaming outside influences. If you have to curtail your workout it will still be better than doing nothing. If you have to run in the rain or train at the gym at the busiest time – you'll just have to grin and bear it if you are to progress positively.

Will it hurt?

It shouldn't, if you do it right.

Working hard will bring rewards but resist the temptation of saying to your body "I'll teach you to get sloppy and out of shape – you're for it now!" This approach is unreasonable. Short, easy sessions will suffice initially if you haven't trained much before – steady does it! Gradually increase the intensity and time of your workouts. As for frequency, always allow at least one day a week, initially two, when you do nothing at all. Rest, and the recovery achieved while at rest, are essential. Your fitness benefits do not end when you finish your workout; your body goes on making adaptations which can only be made while you are at rest. Never do the same weight training routine on consecutive days – this is simply retrogressive, quite apart from the soreness issue.

Try not to be too haphazard in your approach; view the week ahead and try to schedule your workouts in a balanced way. For instance, schedule cardio Monday and Wednesday, resistance Tuesday and Thursday, running, cycling or swimming on Saturday or Sunday. I realise this may be a simplification of a training timetable, not allowing for shift-work, unsociable hours, working and so on: however, the onus is on you to arrange your own training into an achievable structure if you want results.

Running

Why should I run?

* It burns fat.

* It is free (once you've bought your shoes).

* It is guaranteed to get you fit/fitter.

* If you are involved in sports which require you to run, such as football, rugby, tennis and so on, it is going to help improve your overall performance.

I intend to start at the very beginning here for the benefit of people who have never attempted distance running or who have considered it beyond their grasp, for whatever reason. Anybody who has been running for some time should step ahead to the "advanced" section.

You may play the occasional social game of football or tennis and feel you are capable of running about comfortably, but you will find that continuous, long running is very different, and you would be advised to start out by considering yourself a beginner.

I should make the distinction between running and jogging by simply observing that jogging is slow-paced running, sometimes referred to as "running with the brakes on". It is only an alternative way of running, in the same way as sprinting is an alternative, except, unlike sprinting, it is patently obvious that jogging can be sustained for an extended period. During extreme exercise, such as sprinting hard, your body can't get oxygen to your muscles as quickly as they need it, so they switch from working aerobically (with oxygen) to anaerobically (without oxygen). How far can you actually run in the absence of oxygen? In the "advanced" running section you might get the chance to find out!

Newcomers would do well to start out jogging (at about 10-12 minutes a mile) and then step up the pace to 7-9 minute miles; for the first few runs you may even have to slow to walking pace, just until you adjust to the continuity of jogging/running. Don't be discouraged if you struggle on your first few runs. Trust me – it gets better.

When you frequently complete the same run, keep a log of how long it took each time and start to look for small improvements. Do take into account weather conditions, however. Nobody is going to beat their last personal best with a strong wind against them.

To pinpoint your speed, establish a run with a distance of 2-3 miles (preferably in a traffic-free and thus uninterrupted environment, like a park or towpath), clock your run and then do the simple mathematics. Write your speed down each time.

Stretching and Mobilisation

Years ago, we would hold stretches, especially those of the calf muscles, hamstrings and quads for 10-15 seconds each, unaware that we were in some instances doing more harm than good. Hard stretching of cold muscles is a recipe for causing microtrauma – small but painful tears in the muscle.

First of all, it is important to warm the muscles up in a way related to the exercise to follow. Bouncing on the spot, gentle jogging on the spot, bringing the heel up as if to backheel your own backside, and swinging and circling the arms should do the job. After a few minutes of these exercises gently stretch the quads, hamstrings and calves.

When you come to the end of a session, remember to perform a 'cooldown'. When finishing your run, slow down to the slowest jog possible for 400 or so yards and eventually to walking pace for 100-150 yards. Never run flat out and come to a sudden and abrupt halt – always taper off to a slow-paced finish, giving your body a chance to return to its normal state gradually.

A full body stretch, each stretch held for 30 seconds, is advisable to rid the muscles of potentially painful waste products and assist in a full recovery from your exertion.

TOP ROW: HAMSTRINGS; HAMSTRINGS; QUADS.   BOTTOM ROW: QUADS; CALVES.

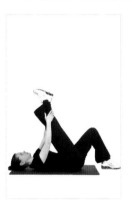 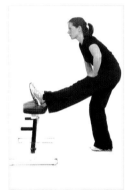 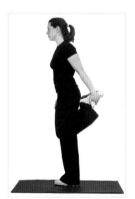

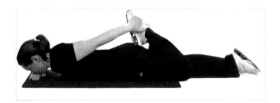

Warm up as you go

Once you have commenced your run, start out by walking briskly, then jogging gently, before hitting

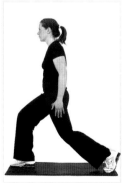

your running stride. Often seasoned runners like to "warm up as you go", gradually increasing the tempo after about 5 minutes of slower running.

Try for 10-15 minutes on your first "full" run, after you have warmed up by walking-jogging. If you run from home, simply run 5-8 minutes, turn around and come back. The suggested increment generally used is to increase the mileage by 10 per cent each time. Alternatively, add another 10 per cent in minutes to your running time (easier to work out than distance).

Technique

I hesitate to advise on running technique, since running should be as natural as walking. When we were children we needed to be taught how to ride a cycle, but nobody had to teach us to run: it was spontaneous. To quote Springsteen, we are "Born to Run".

The few points I would make are:

» Keep your head up. A "head down" style is likely to give you backache. It tends to be common among ex-service personnel who grew used to running with a large pack on their back. Keep your head in line with your spine and your shoulders over the hips. Avoid leaning forward too much; a little should be OK as running bolt upright is, for most, uncomfortable and unnatural. Try to look 20-40 yards ahead with the occasional glance down to avoid obstacles such as tree roots, or, when pavement running, treading in something odious.

» Relax! A relaxed, loping style, free of tension, will make your running easy when you first start. With your arms bent at the elbow let them swing forward effortlessly to and fro in sync with each step, with your hands and wrists completely loose.

» Above all, do what suits you. I have encountered people running marathons with flapping arms, high knee raise and think, "how can they run like that?" But they are obviously doing their own thing, and are happy with it. Try to establish a style that feels natural and comfortable rather than attempting, in the early days, to stylise your technique or copy experienced runners – be yourself.

Advanced

Seasoned runners should look to get out 2-3 times a week for 30+ minutes with one long run of 60 minutes or more, rather than stay in the 30 minute comfort zone the beginners are looking to attain. It will also be beneficial if one of the runs involves an uphill element, and you can fit in a session of interval training (see below). Always try to beat your previous best time to ensure positive progress: if you keep doing the same run at the same pace it will cause your fitness to plateau. Try to challenge yourself on each run.

Interval Training

Competent and experienced runners' training can be supplemented – for running improvement, fitness and as a diversion – by interval training.

This will involve short bursts of sprinting combined with intervals of walking or slow jogging for the purpose of recovery. At first the recovery can be completely passive, simply standing and regaining your breath for the next sprint.

Start out with short runs of 20-30 yards and gradually build up to greater distances, unless you are using this to improve your speed for a specific sport such as football: a midfield player should work on distances from 10-25 yards of speedwork (the training benefit of long runs will provide stamina).

When it comes to speed we are either the beneficiaries or prisoners of our ancestors, who will have unwittingly determined if we will have fast-twitch muscles (for speed) or slow-twitch muscles (for endurance). Everybody has both types of muscle but some, usually the quicker ones, have more fast twitch muscle and often the realisation of this at a young age shapes an individual's athletic prowess. Those with predominately slow-twitch can, fortunately, still improve their speed by training the muscle fibres referred to as 'FOG' (fast oxidative glycolic) with interval training.

I have to be brutally honest at this point and state that interval training means you will have to push yourself really hard to attain significant progress. It will require a little "mind over matter". The choice will be yours – how bad do you want it?

Check for progress by getting a training partner to time your runs. Another way to help improvement is to race against somebody you know to be faster than yourself. I found I never had to look too far…

What if I feel self-conscious?

Too many people have this misconception that if they set off from home for a run, or run by busy roads, people will consider them foolish. Admittedly, some people will consider such activity dumb – after all, they figure "why run if you own a car?" "Because you own a car," is the answer; being continually seated at the wheel of a car will not improve the quality of your heart and the size of your lungs (quite the contrary in fact), but more likely the size of your butt. Most critics, especially people who comment from the windows of their vehicles, are a) morons b) jealous, knowing anything of that nature is beyond their capability c) hapless optimists who presume inactivity is the way to go. You will not look dumb – you will look like somebody trying to improve his health and physique. Just reiterate this view to yourself if doubts creep in. You will find that true friends will agree with you.

Just bite the bullet and get out there, and let them all gaze at your new-found courage and increasing fitness with a mixture of admiration and envy.

I get bored – can I wear my iPod?

If you are running in the park or on a trail in an area that is crime-free I see no problem with this. If you are on a treadmill facing a brick wall it is actually recommended – to stop you losing the will to live. Leave the iPod or mp3 player at home if there is traffic (getting knocked down by an articulated lorry will not be a great start to your running career), or if the area has a dubious reputation. I find it sad but true to relate that I know of at least two people who have been mugged through the inattention created by wearing headphones. They did not hear the approach of their assailants, who were only too aware of this fact. A high-end iPod is a tempting item to the unscrupulous vermin that prey on the trusting and unsuspecting. In such areas leave your valuables at home, including jewellery and expensive watches. I have run in areas like this for years and nobody has wanted to fight me for my Casio to this day.

Leaving your mobile phone at home is advisable unless you are going off on what could be tricky terrain in the middle of nowhere. Never take this hazard on by yourself; there is safety in numbers if even the remotest likelihood of accidents seems a possibility. A sprained ankle in the middle of nowhere is not the most enjoyable experience and even worse if you are by yourself. For a run round the park a phone is just unnecessary baggage, especially if you get time-wasters bothering you with unwanted calls about reducing your bills and so on.

Some more safety points

Try to let somebody know where you will be going if it's not just your usual jaunt around the park and you expect to be out much longer than you usually would. I would also advise that you carry enough small change to make use of a public phone box if you don't want the hassle of having your mobile with you; a few years ago when mobiles were the size and almost the weight of a house brick it would have been akin to weight training but now they are the size of a matchbox it is not impractical. A fellow runner who was resuming training after injury and concerned about a relapse used to carry a bank-note under the innersole of his shoe. "Oh no – not the Achilles again – taxi!"

Beware of the dog (and the bike)

Have you noticed how certain dogs like to chase moving objects? Pigeons, cats, cars and, of course, runners all present an irresistible challenge to them. I like dogs and, until my own dog sadly passed away, I was an owner for fourteen years, but when a dog is coming toward you I advocate making a broad sweep even if the owner looks like a mature, responsible individual and the mutt looks docile – appearances can be deceptive when hounds are involved. If the beast is off the leash, be extremely wary. I have personally been nipped in the ankle by a Dachshund (on Hampstead Heath) and bowled over by a huge friendly-looking Airedale while crossing a narrow footbridge. Both owners, curiously, made the same observation: "Well, he's never done that before!" – implying, I felt, that I had contributed in some manner to the assault and should be apportioned my share of the blame. Always give the loose cur a wide berth, and don't take the attitude "I've got as much right to the footpath as any dog has." Move over. Discretion is the better part of valour in this case. While keeping your wits about you, always be alert to the fast and unheralded arrival of another threat to runners – the adult pavement cyclist. (Kids, I can accept, should be allowed to cycle on the pavement.) Having already decided to break the law by riding on an area designated for pedestrians they appear to now have also assumed right of way – be watchful in areas known for this practice.

Beware of the dark

Never run through ill-lit areas or, worse still, darkened areas, even if you are familiar with the course ahead. I made this mistake and missed the edge of the kerb in the gloom on a rural road I had been running on weekly, and sprained my ankle; going a couple of miles with an ankle growing to the size of a basketball is no fun at all. The safety aspect is obvious if it is an urban area, too.

Running weather, or whether not to...

I would not advocate anybody running in foul weather. If the outlook is for fog, snow, sleet, hail or worse – give it a miss, and go for the treadmill if you can. Never run on icy or snow-covered pavements.

Running in the rain is something I find pleasant and many people who compete will tell you the rain is refreshingly welcome as a coolant – unless it's torrential, of course. If you have decided you will not be deterred by the rain, it may be wise to dress for it by slipping on some light waterproof clothing. (See What to Wear, page 38.)

Running with company

If you feel you would be better off running with somebody for company, and cannot persuade friends, family or colleagues to join you, then a running club could be the answer. A club will make a wealth of information available to you and usually place you in a group to suit your speed and ability. First, establish the club is not solely for elite and/or competing runners and check whether you might find the pace too hot, in more ways than one. Ask questions, be honest about your ability, find out what distances club runs are over and, of course, ascertain the fees involved. It is most likely you will meet people in exactly the same position as yourself that you can run with in comfort, both with the club and at other times that suit you all.

A regular running buddy can be a boon, but be prepared to go solo on the inevitable occasions they "just can't make it", otherwise it becomes an easy excuse to dodge the run yourself and feel justified in blaming somebody else!

If you can't find anybody to keep you company, why not look online? The last time I punched in "running clubs", Google listed 181,000 entries.

Do I need a "special" diet?

Not when you first start running, but if you get serious you may want to consider which foodstuffs are going to be beneficial. A good start is to wave goodbye to junk food; you may have got by on it while living a sedentary lifestyle but now your training will require increased levels of energy and this kind of intake will not come up to the nutritional level you will need.

Get a jump start with a decent breakfast. Even if you don't intend to run until the evening, breakfast is of paramount importance. Porridge, cereal, fruit or wholemeal toast will do the job. If you honestly crave a fat-rich fry-up, try to limit it to once a week. You should be getting stuck into carbohydrates (which provide 50 percent of energy during tough workouts) much more than fats. Try to incorporate pasta, rice and potatoes (not fried) into your meals, combining them with lean chicken and fish as often as possible.

Don't eat a heavy meal within two hours of a long run. Not everybody takes the same time to digest a meal and some foods don't sit too well even if eaten an hour or so before a run (apples in my case). Home in on something you can be pretty sure will not be likely to "make a comeback"; cereals, cereal bars and bananas I have found suit most people I have trained. Keep away from anything fatty or greasy as these are most likely to reappear during your run.

Where to run?

Most of us have little choice but to run on the road, not living by the beach, sandy trail-ways or close to a huge parkland. If you actually do reside in such an area, consider yourself fortunate and make the most of it. This is not to say great runs cannot be found in urban environments. The finest place for running I have encountered is Hampstead Heath in North London, just four miles from central London, with 790 acres of parkland including hills, dales, sandy paths, monstrous climbs and some of the most wonderful scenery a runner could enjoy. If pounding the local granite pavement is a grind, it is often worthwhile, if you can, to jump in the car and drive to a park to get a nice change of scenery and terrain.

If you live in an area where the pavements are comprised of tarmac, or the communications cable layers have recently left a soft tarmac path, take full advantage of it; tarmac is a great surface to run on. A hypermarket car park on a summer evening, or after dark if it's well-lit, makes a reasonable, if less than stimulating, jogging track. Sometimes you just have to settle for uninspiring surroundings when seeking a suitable surface, which is probably why my usual run is to circle an industrial estate.

Don't run dry

Unless you want to hump a water bottle around with you (I recently saw somebody running with a plastic 1 litre bottle and thought "that can't feel comfortable"), drink some water a short while before your run to stay hydrated. If you find on your fledgling runs your mouth becomes dry then try what I prefer, and pop a few mints, such as Polos, in your pocket to refresh you.

What to wear

1. Shoes

Your major outlay will be your footwear. Running shoes for running are as essential as football boots for football, such is their specificity. Those Inter squash shoes may be incredibly comfortable and may have acquired old-friend status but if you run over a mile in them you will learn to regret it. Nothing short of agony lies in wait for the ill-shod runner.

It is vital to purchase your shoes from a recommended, good quality running goods shop, who sell only running-specific equipment. I have used *Runners Needs* and *City Runner* and have found both to be excellent (I have shares in neither).

Run and Become are popular with friends, and if you don't know where to find such a store lash out on a copy of one of the highly informative magazines on running, such as *Runner*, *Runner's World* and *Masters Athletics* (which is aimed at the older but fit runner). These magazines list wholesalers for you to hunt down in your quest for the perfect shoe.

The shops I have mentioned, and, I imagine, all quality running shops, will ask a few pertinent questions before offering you shoes to try on. They will ask how long you have been running, what mileage you expect to do and, of course, your price range. They should then look at your current shoes. Always turn up in trainers; the wear pattern is to an experienced running shoe salesperson the equivalent of a fingerprint to a forensic investigator. You will usually be asked to try a pair on and then run on a treadmill while they video your gait, or as the guy at *Runners Needs* preferred, "run to the phone box and back, mate." He never got it wrong; all these assistants are experienced runners. They know a satisfied customer will return time and time again, and the more they run the more pairs of shoes they will wear out!

I am aware it can be cheaper to buy from mail order or online but getting a proper fitting is paramount to determine if you have normal feet, flat feet, high arches and how much your foot rolls as you land, referred to as pronation.[†] If you are informed you are an 'over-pronator' don't feel offended, it simply means how your foot lands and tells the assistant just what shoe you need. All top brands cater for 'normal' and 'over' pronation as well as 'supination[‡]'; thus informed, the assistant can find out how to tackle any problems by finding the right shoe. Do not be surprised if he also advises you to go a half-size larger in running shoes than your 'street' shoes, as your feet are going to expand with the heat of running and too-tight running shoes can be the source of increasingly excruciating torture.

Different manufacturers use varying materials to try to achieve success in a very competitive market, using gel capsules, kinetic wedges, air capsules and all manner of rocket science-sounding materials. This is why professional advice is required when faced with the dazzling array of features.

---

†   Pronation: The foot lands and twists inwards

‡   Supination: The foot lands and twists outwards

Always lace your shoes in a criss-cross pattern rather than "straight-laced" as it gives a firmer grip. For a totally secure snug fit go for loop-lacing lock (as recommended by *Runners World* magazine), whereby once you have reached the last (top) hole, re-enter the lace back through the same hole until it leaves a loop on each side of the shoe. Then slip the end of the laces through the loop, each to the opposite side, pull them tight and double-knot them. If you have a high instep do the same but miss out one or two pairs of holes on the highest part. Experiment with different ways of lacing until you find which way is

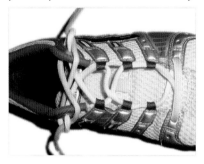

satisfactory for you. Some of this might appear a lot of fiddling about but having to stop to re-tie your laces is an unnecessary irritant which will disrupt your run.

However, be warned – once you've got those shoes on you may succumb to the disease known as "new-shoe syndrome", an irresistible urge to set off on a long test flight.

Look after your shoes

If your shoes are caked in mud it is best to clean them before the mud "bakes" on. Resist the temptation to pop them in the washing machine as it can ruin them. I'm afraid it's a bucket of soapy water and a scrubbing brush. Leave them to dry, but not on the radiator. I always leave mine in the airing cupboard and they have never seemed to suffer for it.

Replacing your shoes

Don't wait until your shoes are completely knackered to replace them. Source their replacement and wear the new ones occasionally to adjust to them. If your shoes are starting to look knackered it is fair to assume they *are* knackered. Running in shoes that are completely played out will only prove detrimental – let's face it, they've probably done 500-700 miles. They deserve to be put to rest.

Do I need any special gear (now I've spent a fortune on my shoes?)

Not really. It might be a good idea to splash out on some running socks. These are designed, unlike general sports socks, to actually move sweat away from your feet and have cushioning in the places you are most likely to need it. This is quite important: the problem most newcomers to running have is blisters caused by chafing socks. Buy them when you get your shoes to check for compatibility, and therefore comfort.

As you progress you might opt for some high-tech running gear composed of 'wicking' fabric, designed to soak up and evaporate sweat; you will see labels advertising the wonders of Dri-fit, Clima Lite, Cool Max. They all appear to do what it says on the label and the quality of the garments is indisputable. Alternatively, when starting out, you can do what has suited most people prior to the advent of these wonder garments and slip on a comfortable, well-washed cotton t-shirt. Bear in mind that a sweat-drenched t-shirt will be unlikely to enhance the quality of your run and you may want, in time, to consider switching to a material that will wick away sweat. Never wear a box-fresh cotton top, and, while you may want to declare your undying love and devotion to Leyton Orient or Partick Thistle, that nylon replica shirt is inadvisable running wear as well. Tops such as the afore-mentioned can bring about the dreaded blood-drawing "joggers' nipple", which is no laughing matter. If you are unsure whether seams appear likely to chafe vulnerable body parts, play it safe and smear any suspect regions with petroleum jelly (Vaseline).

The same goes for shorts. Keep away from the shiny nylon football shorts variety (I've seen them draw blood from the inside of somebody's thigh) and opt for cotton or polyester. Ditto for track trousers. Popular with serious runners are close-fitting, purpose-made leggings such as the now legendary Ron Hill tracksters. From a purely personal point of view I prefer something just a little more roomy with a zip pocket for my front door key.

Somebody may have suggested that wearing bin-liners under your clothing is a sure-fire way of burning fat. Be warned – this is more likely to dehydrate you. They are fine as a heat retainer for the first half mile of a marathon (where you spend most of the time shuffling due to the crowded start) until the experienced runners get warmed up, but could prove dangerous to the novice runner.

Waterproofs are a good investment. The thin variety from budget sports shops will suffice in the early days, but as you run more and more you may want to invest in a garment that is completely waterproof and windproof, but breathable.

In cold weather you will need a hat. This is where you can declare your undying devotion to West Brom or whoever as any old hat will pretty much do the job. It may be you suffer from cold hands in low temperatures. Some people do so more so than others; if this is the case, slip some gloves on – again, cheap and cheerful will do the job.

Gadgets

Watch

A digital watch, preferably with a stopwatch facility, is really all you need to start with. You will not need Tag or Rolex for your timekeeping – Casio or Timex will do equally well. Most "sports" watches, even the budget variety, have a countdown facility and a "lap counter" to record your running history. A backlight for those running in the hours of darkness has an obvious benefit.

Pedometers

A low-tech device (the lower-tech the better in my estimation) to tell you how many steps you have taken and thus, by a (hopefully) simple deduction, how far you have actually travelled. A short while ago a well-known cereal manufacturer was giving these away with a packet of its produce. You can get a version that will record your previous runs; others combine time and date, stopwatch, radio and panic alarm. Some will even talk to you, and there are wireless models that claim 98% accuracy. There are versions that are interactive and can have their information downloaded into your computer. At this point I would like to comment that I have had a computer crash on me, but never a desk diary – my favourite storage device for my exertions – but to each his own.

While the model you invest in may lack NASA-standard accuracy, it will at least be consistent for every one of your individual performances, showing you if you have travelled further or faster.

Treadmills

Some people only ever run on treadmills, such is their disdain for road running. What I have tried in the following is to give the best and worst points of treadmill usage. I personally prefer road running but don't mind the treadmill, especially considering how sophisticated they have become. If you find the initial sensation of running on a treadmill strange, try the lowest elevation setting, which may offer a more natural feel. You can buy 'home' versions but you should first enquire about:

- the weight of the machine

- the strength of your floor

- the quality of the machine – most gym machines are of vastly superior quality both in engineering and performance to home machines, but you may need a solid floor and an unlimited budget.

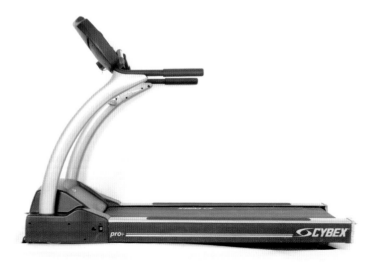

Reading

There are a myriad of running books but Jeff Galloway's *Running: Getting Started* (2005) Meyer & Meyer Sports Books is a great one to kick off with, as is *Running Made Easy* by S. Whalley (2004) Robson Books. Also *Running: Fitness and Injuries, A Self Help Guide* by Vivian Grisogond (John Murray).

Runners World and *Runner* magazines are full of hard-headed, sensible information and tips; they give tests and ratings for shoes and apparel to give readers an informed choice. They give listings of races, from "fun runs" to marathons. I recommend both publications.

Cycling

Cycling, whether indoors on a static cycle or on the open road, will provide excellent cardiovascular exercise. Both versions are beneficial for the heart, lungs, for helping to lower cholesterol and for cardiovascular endurance. Fat burning potential, however, is not as great, compared over the same period of time, and with equal exertion, to running, rowing and using the cross-trainer. To obtain positive fitness progress as an outdoor cyclist, especially if your route involves traffic that forces a "stop, go" routine, you will need a lengthy time in the saddle which, for obvious reasons, achieves better results than cycling with lots of pauses.

It is with this in mind I have focused on static cycles wherein exercise can be organised into a continuous workout. The disadvantages are the lack of fresh air and the boredom factor; to combat the latter either set up in front of the TV or wear a portable audio device, preferably one that will provide stimulating music. The advantages are numerous. Access is easy – all the big gyms have a plentiful supply of up-to-date exercise bikes.

» Static cycles give instant feedback regarding speed, distance, heart rate, calorific expenditure, wattage and many are compatible with major brands of heart rate monitors to ensure you are working in your desired training zone.

» You do not need any special motor skills or enhanced co-ordination capability as exercise bikes are foolproof. If you can't ride an upright bike due to back problems you should seek out a recumbent cycle.

» No articulated lorries will be threatening your life and you won't need any specific gear or clothing. You are unlikely to have to leave your bike unattended for five minutes only to return and find it stolen.

» If the amount of impacting or pounding-type exercise you are doing is having a negative effect, substitute cycling as it is kind to the hips, knees and ankles, as well as the hamstrings and calf muscles.

Workouts

Most gym bikes offer a range of settings such as manual (use this until you get used to the machine), hill climb, random, incline, race and even more. Picking one bike at random, the Reebok 5 Series, aimed at the home market, offers 10 programmes and 10 levels of resistance. Whatever bike you are using, try all the programmes to see which suit your purpose.

If you are training at home on a basic machine then alternate long endurance sessions of 30-40 minutes with interval training. This does not have to be complicated. Start with this easy routine:

• Cycle easy for 5 minutes to warm up.

• Cycle hard for 1 minute, then easy for 2 minutes. Repeat for 20-30 minutes.

When this becomes too easy (after your warm-up):

• Cycle hard for 5 minutes, then easy for 5 minutes. Repeat for 30 minutes.

• Change the intervals as you see fit but keep the "hard" sessions and "easy" sessions proportionate. It won't pay to get too top-heavy with either.

• Always have a cool-down stretch after a long session on the bike, just as you would following a run.

Thinking of buying an exercise bike? Some points to consider:

» *Display console.* All new bikes have a display console but check it out before buying to establish if it is comprehensive enough for your needs, and large enough to read at a glance – unless you intend to always train wearing your reading spectacles.

» *Weight tolerance.* Big boys beware! Cheaper models often have an upper weight limit of 16 stones.

» *Size.* Do you have adequate room? Upright cycles are not too demanding on space but recumbent cycles tend to be space hogs, in addition to being more expensive.

» *Assembly.* Does it come ready-assembled or will you need to call on your DIY skills? How tricky is it to put together? The beauty of a second-hand model is that somebody has already carried out the (often painstaking) construction work.

» *Saddle comfort.* Check the saddle for comfort. This will not be something you will want to find out, literally, the hard way. Some have a gel saddle – a point worth considering if comfort in this area is an issue.

» *Noise.* Air braking is where wind resistance is utilised by the provision of a large fan. One bonus is that it provides a cooling blast of air up your hot legs (even if it does take a bit of getting used to), but the noise level with most of these models is pretty high. Electronic braking is the most common system in use and along with mechanical breaking is quiet when in use.

» *Quality of ride.* Electronic braking gives the smoothest ride, but is the most expensive. Mechanical braking is adequate but needs a substantial flywheel (controlled by magnets) for a reasonable action; the bigger the flywheel, preferably made of steel, the smoother the ride. This version is likely to need some minor mechanical attention from time to time.

» *Second-hand.* Those free newspapers that are usually recycled unread, or the local press, usually have a wealth of second-hand exercise bikes. If you choose to buy second-hand, take a good look over the bike first, and try it out. Some years ago I bought what seemed like a reasonable-looking second-hand bike, but on getting it home found that, although it functioned adequately, its action was as loud as a building-site generator. Try before you buy, whether new or used.

Spinning bikes

Spinning classes have become a common feature of most major gyms. You need a reasonable level of fitness to do these classes as they can be physically demanding, but should result in a high level of fitness if attended regularly. A word of warning: I found the experience of sitting on the saddle something akin to sitting on a large, dull knife-blade. As you are up and out of the saddle, peddling for all you're worth for much of the time, you don't have to endure it for long periods. They are a relatively small, nice-looking piece of equipment and fine for home use, but try that saddle out first…

Rowing Machines

I admit to being a major fan of rowing machines. Organised and structured workouts on a rowing machine provide the following benefits:

» Improves aerobic activity

» Improves muscle tone and uses every major muscle group (Fluid Rower actually claim 84% of muscles are used)

» Improves stamina

» Weight bearing and impact free (no jarring of joints)

» Ideal for older or heavier-built people

» Excellent for rehabilitation i.e. those with knee problems

» Great as a component of a cross-training regime, combining well with running and cycling

» Usually plentiful at gyms (I've rarely seen them all in use at the same time, unlike some other cardiovascular equipment). Suitable for home use and compared to the cost of some other home equipment, competitively priced, even with a high end machine such as Concept II, the most popular at under £1000. A quick search on eBay revealed 23 various models for sale with a general price of around £300-£400. The Concept and the Fluid Rower can both be folded or stood on end to take up less space. Fully extended, they measure 7-8 feet.

I should balance my admiration for the machine with what may be considered drawbacks:

» Back pain sufferers should take professional advice to ensure that their use of a rowing machine will not aggravate an existing condition (although, for the majority of people, these machines are terrific for strengthening the back).

» The need to develop correct technique to gain full benefit. I have witnessed some dire technique but any capable instructor should be able to rectify this in a matter of minutes. The most common complaint is similar to that expressed about running and static cycling – that of tedium. Some folk find it boring to slide to and fro for 20-30 minutes at a stretch. My advice (as with static cycling): park yourself in front of the TV, or get yourself an mp3 player or iPod in a purpose built clip-on case or armband.

» If you have dashed out and with all good intentions bought yourself a Concept, Fluid Rower or Water Rower and have now tired of it, they make an expensive and space-hogging ornament/clothes horse.

A rowing machine in the garage or spare room is ideal for home training, but before you actually buy one:

• Try one at the local gym when they have an open or "tester" day, or get a friend to take you as a guest.

• Measure the available space (weight is irrelevant as the heaviest models weigh under 11 stones).

- Check out the after-sales reputation and warranty.

- See if the instrumentation panel will give you what you are looking for. Get one you can see clearly, especially if you don't want to train wearing spectacles. Instrumentation is important to "log" your progress and get instant feedback.

- Check how comfortable the seat feels (I have seen people insert a folded towel under their backside for comfort) and imagine how comfortable it will feel after 30 minutes or more. Does the sliding action feel smooth and reassuring? You don't want to spend your workout like a rodeo rider waiting for the bell.

  Before you take a seat…

  » Tie shoe laces and draw-strings on shorts or track bottoms securely. The only real risk in rowing is getting a dangling shoelace trapped in the sliding mechanism (a major embarrassment if occurring at the gym).

  » Easy on the jewellery – rings can scrape against the handle or adjoining finger, which can irritate or cause blisters.

  » Don't go barefoot! Comfortable trainers, properly laced, are essential.

  » After 30 minutes it is not unusual to be a little saddle-sore and feel that your backside has "gone to sleep". Padding may be the answer, but (if this is the case) I favour stopping every 10-15 minutes (there is a "rest" facility on the Concept Rowers), sip some water and stretch the glutes (abbreviation of *gluteus maximus* = buttock muscles) briefly before resuming the workout. This will have little, if any, detrimental bearing on your overall exercise.

  » As mentioned, if the boredom factor is becoming problematic, turn on the TV or hi-fi, or, if you're at the gym, a portable audio device. I tend to turn my own iPod up louder than I should simply to drown out the gym's music or irksome stentorian mobile phone users; mobile phone usage is mercifully banned at the gym where I instruct unless somebody is expecting an urgent call regarding a birth, or a pools win.

Technique

Are you sitting comfortably?

If you are using a machine for the first time, ensure the foot setting is right for you and the straps are snug but not too tight. Check this by sliding to and fro a few times before grasping the handle (some manufacturers refer to it as "the oar"). Remember – if it doesn't feel comfortable at this stage, it isn't likely to improve from here on in.

Resistance setting

The following refers to the Concept Rowers as you are most likely to come across this brand at the gym.

On the side of the drum (metal on older versions, plastic on new ones) which contains the fan is a lever, calibrated from 1-10. Number 1 is the easiest setting, and the higher you go the more the dampener is employed to increase resistance, making 10 the hardest setting.

It is not the case that the higher the setting the more you will derive from the workout. People aiming mainly at weight reduction should try using a heart rate monitor and work between 60-70% of their maximum heart rate, starting out on setting 4-5, increasing by one setting higher whenever this becomes easy. Work on the rower, as with all equipment, needs to be a little challenging to bring about progress.

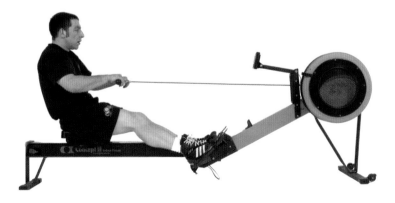

The Return Position, The Catch, The Drive, The Finish

1. The Return

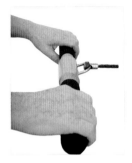

You should be comfortably seated with your hands hooked over the rubber handles of the "oar". Your grip should be light but firm, as opposed to clenching tightly. Your wrists should remain 'flat', as pictured. The chain is parallel to the floor – keep it that way in the stages to follow, and don't allow it to elevate or dip.

2. The Catch

Keeping the chain parallel to the floor, move your upper body forward, bending at the knees until your lower legs are perpendicular to the floor. Keep your head up and prepare for the drive backward.

3. The Drive

Pull the oar towards you as you slide backwards, propelled by extending your legs. Keep your arms long until the oar passes over the knees. Keep your back straight and your head up.

4. The Finish

Your legs straighten out as the oar is pulled to the waist; your elbows should be drawn back past the body with the lower arms parallel to the floor and wrists kept flat. Keep your back straight as you lean back slightly at the conclusion, before returning to position one, the Return.

Do not:

✗ Whip the chain toward you – simply pull it evenly and smoothly.

✗ Go off line – keep the chain parallel to the floor.

✗ Pull the oar to the chest – too high: pull to the waistline.

✗ Raise the knees prematurely, forcing you to flip the chain to clear them.

✗ Use your back to achieve the drive – using your legs is vital.

✗ Bend your wrists – keep them flat. Twist the chain.

✗ Forget to replace the oar in its holster.

✗ Forget to adjust the resistance lever before getting "strapped in", as you will have to undo the straps and dismount to do so.

Rowing Programmes

• After a short stretch, row easily for 5 minutes to warm you up on 25 strokes per minute.

• If you have never used the machine before, progress to a 10 minute session on level 4 and increase your time by 2 minutes each time until 20 minutes at level 5 becomes comfortable.

Then:

• On setting 5, row for 20 minutes at 28-30 strokes per minute.

Then:

• On setting 6, row for 30 minutes at 30-32 strokes per minute.

Then:

• The same as above but try to increase the distance you cover, or the calories you burn if weight loss is your aim.

Since this section assumes you're using a Concept rowing machine, let's look at the advice the manufacturers give on their website. They state: "The best guideline for weight-loss is to aim for rows of 30 minutes at a comfortably intense pace." Eventually, progress to a 45 minute session of varying speeds on setting 7-10 at least once a week, combined with interval training of:

• 3-5 minutes easy (25-30 strokes per minute)

• Alternating with: 3-5 minutes fast (30-40 strokes per minute)

Moving on

Concept's website enables you to download training plans which are suitable for any rowing machine. It also has a training forum.

Group rowing classes are gaining popularity in gyms; an instructor calls the shots while everybody lines up on their rowers to toil at the commands. Worth trying once, I feel, but check on the expected fitness level before committing yourself.

After you have completed a lengthy session on the rower, cool down just as you would after a run. (See Stretching, page 143.) Indoor rowing competitions have become commonplace, with results published regularly in *Ultrafit Magazine* (which often gives advice on improving your rowing). Check the times competitors have posted and see how you measure up against them. Whatever your own results are, of one thing you can be sure – regular rowing machine workouts will help you attain and maintain good physical condition.

Cross-training machines (also known as elliptical trainers)

Particularly handy machines for anybody who has a problem with high impact exercises (such as running and skipping) as its smooth, fluid action is of a very low impact nature, which makes it kind to the knees, calves and ankles. It allows a movement that is a hybrid of running and cross-country skiing.

It requires only basic

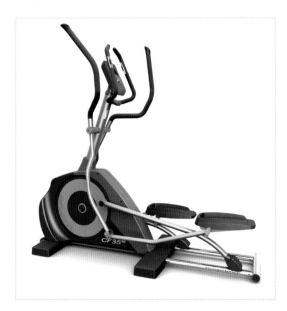

co-ordination skills, but, if you're using one for the first time, start out slow, until you are comfortable with the combined action of arms and legs. There is an alternative set of fixed handles for anybody wanting to use only their legs. Most of these machines have a clear and informative display for checking your heart rate, speed and energy expenditure, as well as a varied choice of training programmes.

Manufacturers promise a high calorific burn of 750 calories an hour or more, but I am never sure of the veracity of these "ballpark" figures on calories expended. It does give a great workout and I recommend it highly as part of a cardiovascular cross-training routine.

Skipping

There are numerous benefits to skipping; if you cannot already skip it is worth taking the time to learn. While there are some exercises it's impractical to learn from a book, skipping isn't one of them; it is, literally, child's play.

Reasons to skip

» Allows aerobic and anaerobic training. You simply decide what level of exertion you want to work at.

» Tones muscle and reduces fat.

» Increases leg power and endurance.

» Improves co-ordination, agility and balance as upper and lower body adapt to the simple harmony required.

» Increases joint strength and, as in most rebounding exercises, improves bone density.

» Beneficial even when used in short intervals; especially efficient as a warm-up or cool-down exercise.

- » A refreshing fitness regime to condition the body for most sports, especially boxing, martial arts and all racquet sports: in other words, those requiring the upper and lower body to synchronize.

- » Provides perfect cross-training benefits for most exercise regimes and sports.

- » You do not have to master "flash" moves and manoeuvres to derive a useful workout. Very basic steps will be sufficient to get results.

- » There is something enjoyable in performing an exercise that is improved (in my opinion) by using music to assist your sense of rhythm.

Usual reasons put forward for not skipping

- • 'I'm a bit on the clumsy/heavy side.'

- • 'I have poor co-ordination.'

- • 'I'll look stupid.'

I can appreciate these objections and have come across them frequently but I have found that most objectors are often astonished by just how easily and rapidly they become adept at skipping.

Learning a new skill is always rewarding and learning something as simple as skipping, while hardly up there with learning the trapeze, is extremely satisfying, especially if you had elements of doubt. I have taught hundreds of people to skip. Some have taken under a minute, some may have taken a lot longer, but they all have one thing in common – they have all mastered it. I have never, as yet, had a failure, and while some of them will never be mistaken for Floyd Mayweather, they can all skip well enough to get a good workout from it.

Before you make a start there are three major considerations:

- » Length, material and quality of your rope.

- » Surface

- » Footwear.

Ropes

(All skipping materials, whether rope, plastic, wire, leather and so on, are referred to as "ropes".)

When you first start skipping, a light leather or PVC rope will suffice. You may later decide to try out heavy ropes, or those composed of wire, plastic tubing or plastic beads; these ropes make increased demands on you, so kick off with the basic variety.

Whichever rope you settle on it is vital to have it properly sized, as pictured opposite. Ideally, a beginner should have a rope they can stand on with the leading foot, where the handles reach the armpits. Extremely tall people may need to get a "made to measure" bespoke version. Fortunately this involves very little expense: these can be obtained from good sports or martial arts stores, or from the internet. For shorter people it is a simple task to shorten a rope; measure the rope by standing on the centre as before, measure the excess amount, cut it off with scissors or a craft knife and re-secure in the holder by applying a cable tie (available at any DIY store at minimal cost). Err on the longer side at first. You can always cut a little more off – you can't put it back on!

Leather Ropes

Traditional leather ropes usually come with user-friendly wooden handles and can have swivelling or ball-bearings in the handle for a smooth action.

PVC Speed Ropes

Intended, as the name implies, to improve foot speed. They are usually a little cheaper than leather ropes. If trying one for the first time, my tip would be to wear jogging bottoms to minimise "whiplash" on the legs or hindquarters until you become accustomed to the rope.

"Heavy Handed" Ropes

These are designed, or at least this is their intention, to intensify the workout, in particular to the upper body. The handles are hollow and contain small metal bars; not recommended for beginners, but experienced skippers can achieve improved arm strength over a period of time. I would suggest, on first using this kind of rope, to work for short periods and then gradually build up.

Long Handled/ Extendable Ropes

Ropes with a long handle make crossovers and other intricate manoeuvres easier to perform; again, unsuited to beginners.

Cable Ropes

These are made from light, thin strands of metal and can turn incredibly fast for a demanding anaerobic workout. If using them for the first time I would seriously advise against wearing shorts – in case you suffer "the lash", which may deter you from further use. Definitely unsuitable for beginners.

"Thai" Ropes

Popular with Thai boxers, these consist of a "rope" of clear plastic tubing, sold incredibly cheaply in Thailand (a student picked one up for me for the princely sum of fifty pence). These quickly let the user feel the effect on the arms and shoulders and can only be described as hard

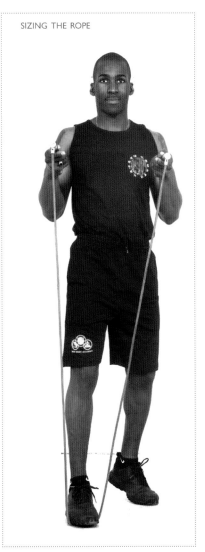

SIZING THE ROPE

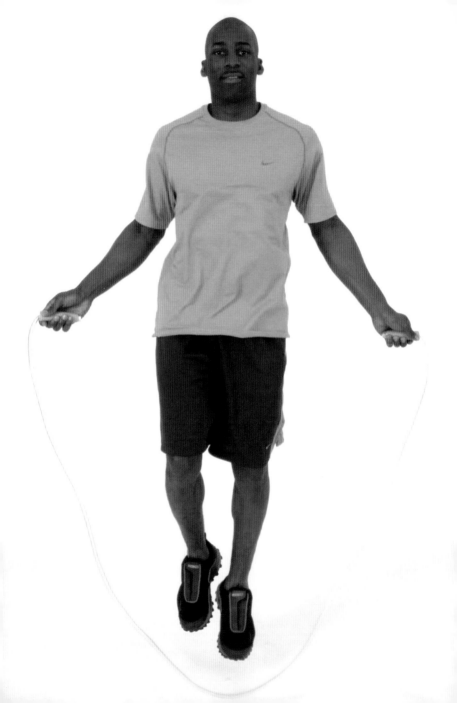

work, but nonetheless rewarding if you can stick with it. Definitely for seasoned skippers only. See picture, left.

Beaded Ropes

Composed of cord covered in plastic beads these are slower on the turns but heavy enough to provide a good all-round workout. Not too bad for beginners as they are slow enough to allow control.

Surface

Do not skip on concrete, tarmac or other hard surfaces. The very least you are likely to suffer are blisters on your feet and sore calf muscles. Ideally you need a sprung wooden floor, or a rubberised gym matted floor. Skipping indoors on carpet is unlikely to prove harmful, but if you have a laminated floor that is perfect.

Footwear

Running, baseball or tennis shoes, cross-training shoes, boxing or wrestling boots are all ideal. Make sure your laces are securely tightened as a trailing lace will halt the rope's progress. If you feel the desire to skip in bare feet I suggest you opt for a judo mat or a carpeted floor.

Other considerations

- Long hair? Tie it back.

- Loose-fitting spectacles? Tie them around the back of the head to avoid watching them take flight across the room.

- You may want to place your drinks bottle nearby to sip between intervals of skipping.

- Skip where you can see the clock (you can't look at your wristwatch) or have a timer with an alarm within hearing range; get a kitchen timer (about £3 in Sainsbury's) or use the stopwatch facility on your mobile phone.

Actually getting started!

Be prepared to be a little patient with yourself at first. It may take a few false starts before you become accomplished. If you have a background in gymnastics, dance or sports it should be easy; if not – don't despair, it's still easy. It may just take a little longer.

Start-up position

Where possible, stand opposite a full-length mirror. It is important to keep your head up, in line with your spine, at all times. In order to maintain a good ergonomic posture, resist the temptation to glance down at your feet to see how they are doing! Regulate your breathing by inhaling deeply through your nose to keep some air in the tank. Initially skipping can be tiring.

Start with feet a little less than shoulder width apart, the rope resting on your calf muscles.

Getting moving

Begin by bouncing lightly on the balls of your feet. Once you have established an easy, effortless bouncing rhythm, flip the rope over your head, clearing your feet by a few inches with each revolution. You will hit your feet from time to time, which can be frustrating just as you think you are getting the hang of it. A good tip when this occurs is to continue bouncing at the same tempo and flip the rope back over your head to the start-up position and then carry on as before; by not stopping and keeping your "bounce" going, it will serve to improve your technique and keep your workout seamless. As you gain confidence, bring your elbows in a little closer to the body, allowing the lower arms to do more of the work.

Again, be patient. Remember when you first learned to drive or ride a bike – this is simple by comparison, and carries relatively less risk of injury.

Moving on

So – you can do the "bouncing on the spot" skip? Let's move on…

Alternate Stepping

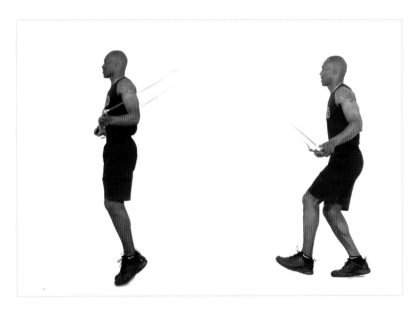

Starting off with the two-footed bounce, progress to placing your feet alternately to the front, as if putting out a couple of lighted cigarette butts! Vary this by taking a double beat with each foot.

Ski Hops

Feet together, hop from side to side, then switch to hopping backward and forward.

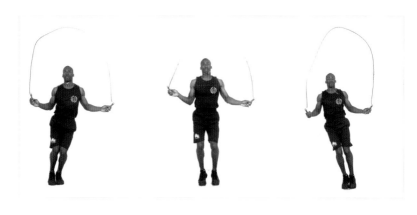

Split Steps

Start with feet together, then as you skip open to shoulder width and back again.

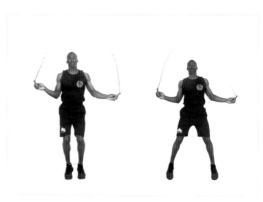

Hop and Kick

Hop on one foot, then take a small kick to the front with the other. The classic-looking "boxing skip".

X-Legged

Start with the bouncing skip, then cross and uncross your feet.

Leg Raise

Work the lower abdominal muscles as you skip! While bouncing on one foot, raise the other leg to form a right angle.

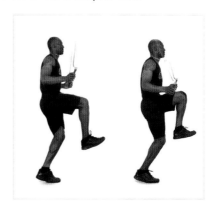

Cross-overs

You will need a longish rope, and the longer the handles the better. Start off by bouncing then cross your arms in front of you, so the rope forms a loop which you pass under your feet with a downward sweep of your crossed arms. Once the rope has passed under your feet, bring your arms back to the start position. At first it will take a little getting used to but think how impressive it will look once you can perform a continuous series of cross-overs like a professional boxer.

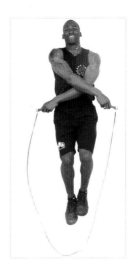

Running in Place

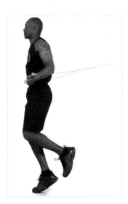

This is where you should be working hard! Run on the spot as you skip, varying the pace but trying to finish with a flat-out burst. If you have a good space to skip in, run forward and backward, or create your own variations on the running theme. If you think running with a skipping rope is demanding, think of the guy who skipped the entire London Marathon a few years ago.

Back and Forth

Run forward a few yards then back up with fast alternating steps, mixing in some "Leg Raise" (see above) running. If space allows, run forward and backward at top speed for short bursts.

Bumps

I've always called these "bumps" (there is probably a more technical term) but I think it explains the action; after bouncing, leap high with raised knees as the rope does a double-spin. See how many you can do continuously until you get that lung-bursting feeling that leaves you in no doubt you are now working anaerobically. This is a good way to finish off a "Running Skip": concluding by beating your previous best "bumps" record.

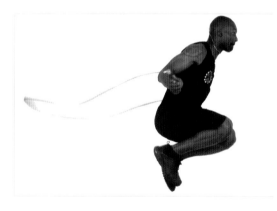

Reverse Skipping

The ultimate skip challenge! Start with the rope resting on your shins and try skipping by turning the rope from front to back. I must admit that this takes a bit of getting used to.

Get Rhythm

Get some upbeat music going, be it techno, hip-hop or good old rock'n'roll to give you a sense of rhythm and alleviate boredom; skipping in silence is soulless and suited exclusively to any Trappist Monk striving for upper and lower body co-ordination.

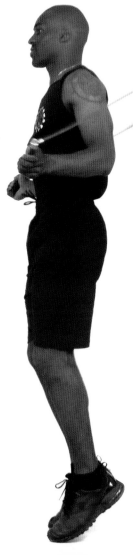

Weights and other resistance training

Weight training

ANY REGIME INTENDED TO GET YOU INTO BETTER shape will almost certainly require some element of resistance training. Simply put, by overloading a muscle you are stimulating it to adapt to the increased load. In the case of most men, due to the presence of the hormone testosterone, the muscle will grow slightly larger, as new muscle fibres are recruited. Men have a much higher level of testosterone than women (it is a steroid androgen formed in the testicles, which may go some way towards explaining the reason why) which is the simple reason men find it easier than women to grow large muscles. There are factors which govern how much and how big your muscles can grow. Heredity plays a part in this; if your ancestors have bestowed to you larger, fast-contracting, fast twitch muscle fibres then muscle growth will be a realistic capability. Do not despair if you are in the slow-twitch group – you are just going to have to work that bit harder to get results. The following is a simplistic explanation of why weight training works.

There are many forms of resistance training. For instance, there is the straightforward press up or push up, where you simply (simpler for some than others) lift your own body weight from the floor. The weight, in this case, is whatever you weigh, but by lifting variable loads it becomes possible to gradually increase the load and, in doing so, increase your strength. This can be achieved by using free weights or machine weights. With free weights you add more plates to a bar or use a larger dumbbell; with machine weights you set the machine to the next level once the current setting is no longer sufficiently demanding.

Why does it work

The simple reason why weight training builds bigger and stronger muscles is, ironically, due to the damage it causes. Lifting weights results in microscopic tears to the muscle fibres. The repair work the body responds with enlarges and increases the amount of fibres. This microscopic tearing is the reason why you will often feel a soreness within 48 hours after lifting, referred to as Delayed Onset Muscle Soreness (DOMS). The best way to deal with this effect is to always cool down properly, stretch – especially the muscle groups you have been working – and rest from resistance training of these muscles for at least 24 hours. If you really want to work 6 days a week (everybody needs one day off), you will need to perform Split Routines (page 82).

Benefits of weight training

- » Builds strength

- » Improves muscular fitness

- » Burns off excess fat (by increasing metabolic rate)

- » Increases bone density

- » Lowers blood pressure

- » Improves posture and appearance

- » Improves sporting fitness (especially when tailored to specific sports).

The "appearance factor" is, I feel, a strong attraction to many who get involved in weight training; it has a knock-on effect, whereby if you start to look better, you start to feel better and renewed self-confidence invariably results.

Learn the correct way

The best way to get started is to receive instruction from a qualified instructor – so much better than a well-intentioned friend or a book. Books to give you inspiration and advice are plentiful and useful, but you must learn the basics first; just as in learning to drive, it is always better to learn from somebody qualified than from a helpful friend or relative. You need a programme that is tailored to you. A good instructor should listen to your personal fitness goals and build them into the plan they draw up for you. If they don't, then find a new instructor! Safety is paramount and only an experienced instructor is guaranteed to point out the way to lift weights safely and confidently. See Safety First below.

When you undertake resistance training, you are faced with the choice between free weights or machine/fixed weights.

Arguments for and against free weights

AGAINST

X   Require professional instruction for safe use (if beginners want to avoid accidents or "overloads").

X   More time-consuming. You have to change plates manually as opposed to moving the pin on machines.

X   When working with very heavy free weights it is important to enlist the aid of a "spotter" – somebody to stand by to assist you should the lift prove beyond your capability, a common occurrence, especially on the closing repetitions of a difficult set. This is an extremely important safety aspect and should never be disregarded. The spotter or, better still, spotters, should keep their hands in close proximity to the weight in order to react swiftly if something is starting to go wrong.

FOR

✓   Versatile.

✓   Suit advanced/experienced trainers.

✓   Encourage motor skills and bilateral strength (with use of dumbbells).

✓   Inexpensive, compared to machine weights.

✓   Ideal for home use, in the shed, garage, spare room or wherever there is a reasonably small space.

Arguments for and against machine weights

AGAINST

✗ Restrict movement to a single, not always natural, plane.

✗ Does not utilise motor skills as much as free weights. Moves can seem robotic.

✗ Expensive: most people could not afford to have a comprehensive set at home.

✗ Space-hogs: machines require a lot of room if installed at home.

✗ Require regular maintenance.

FOR

✓ Safer (with professional instruction).

✓ Practically eliminates the chance of theft.

✓ User-friendly for beginners.

✓ Time-saving, for the majority of exercises.

So, armed with this information, the choice of your strength training lies with either

- Free weights

- Machine weights

- A combination of both.

All newcomers to weight training must be aware of the risks involved. Injury comes easily when there is misuse or complacency regarding safety, and this is why professional tuition is so important – not just for helping you get results, but, just as importantly, helping you avoid injury.

Safety first

Once you have learned to handle weights competently it is worth being aware of the following: If you elect to train at home, keep it as light as possible, especially if you are a novice. Try to train with a partner in order to assist one another by spotting (tracking the movements of weights, or assisting at the start and finish of moves and also being on hand to offer help in case of difficulties).

- If weights need to be held in place by an Allen Key, spring collar or screw-type collar, check they are tight every time you use them. Falling weight discs and soft footwear are not a happy combination.

- Only perform recognised exercises as demonstrated by an instructor or listed in respected manuals. Never attempt to improvise or invent moves of your own.

- Work slowly – this way you will recruit the maximum amount of muscle fibre. You will also have complete control of your equipment, paramount for safety. There are no bona fide exercises that need to be performed hurriedly.

- Always maintain a straight back. The two most common reasons, in my experience, for people packing in weight training are:

  » boredom (they have never changed/upgraded their programme)

  » they hurt their back through bad technique.

- Don't be a hero. This is mainly a macho thing: the guy who preceded you on the machine just lifted 50kg, you don't want to now appear wimpy by shifting down to your prescribed 20kg, so you make a futile and highly ill-advised attempt at 50kg. Don't do this! You may do yourself irreparable harm as you struggle to lift what is obviously an excessive overload. Remember that we all have different needs. Lifting light weights should never be regarded in any way as a sign of inadequacy. It is, in fact, recommended for many aspects of martial arts and boxing training. If you are unsure of which weight to use, aim low; you can always put more weight on, but you can't take it off when you've got the bar stuck at half-way. Just be yourself and do your own thing. Ignore other people's weight volumes and techniques and stick to your own plan.

- Don't copy other people – always stick to the way the instructor has shown you. You may espy somebody working out and be tempted to think "that looks good, I'll try it." This could be disastrous, as the other person is likely to be either using an advanced technique, or, worse still, incorrect technique.

- Be patient. We all progress at different rates. Some people show improvements rapidly, others take months and months. Never despair, it always works if you just give it time.

Machine weights

Once you have been to the gym and learned the safe and sure way to work with weights from a competent instructor, he or she should design a personalised programme for you. For that reason I am providing here a workout designed for the home user who does not have access to machine weights, but which can also be used by gym patrons where there is access to free weights. I have also provided the machine equivalent as I realise many people have built a home gym which may be composed wholly or partly of machines. There are so many varieties of machine weights, and techniques tend to differ according to the manufacturer. For instance, some chest press machines require you to be prone while exercising, while others have you sitting up. For beneficial results you need to be shown, at least initially, how to use the equipment by a qualified instructor. Never jump on a piece of weights machinery if you do not know how to use it properly.

Free weights

I advocate working in the following order. All exercises have one thing in common – *work slowly.*

The following workout is an all-body routine and you *must* rest the following day, to recover and let your muscles adapt. Failure to do so is likely to result in a great deal of soreness.

(see Split Routines, page 82.)

> ~Tip~
> Breathing; exhale on the exertion, or use this crude but effective mantra – "blow on the effort".

All weights workouts should be preceded with a warm-up – ideally 5 minutes of cardiovascular exercise, joint mobility and a short stretch (6-8 seconds per body part). The workout should then be followed by a cool down – at least 5 minutes of cardiovascular exercise, then a long stretch (20-30 seconds per body part).

This is a very basic "10 Rep Max Workout", which is to say the first repetition is easy but by the tenth that last repetition should be challenging (but never painful). If it hurts – stop, before you cause harm. Always be certain you are capable of lifting the weight you intend to work with.

Exercise	Reps
Dumbell flyes	10
Bench Press	10
Single Arm Dumbbell Rows	10
Upright Rows	10
Front Raise	10
Dumbell Shoulder Press	10
Seated bent-over lateral raise	10
Barbell or Dumbbell Squats	10
Deadlift	10
Dumbbell Bicep Curls	10
Single Arm Seated Triceps Extensions	10

1. Dumbbell Flyes (Chest exercise)

Lay on a flat weights bench; if you are improvising at home, ensure the bench allows unrestricted shoulder movement. Hold the dumbbells directly above your shoulders while maintaining a slight bend in your arms. Lower your arms out to the sides, level with the chest, pause for 1-2 seconds then return to the start point. This exercise targets the pectoral muscles and serves to pre-exhaust the chest prior to the bench press (see below.)

⇨ *Machine equivalent: 'Pec Deck Flyes'*

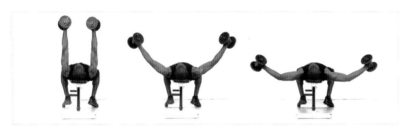

2. Bench Press (chest exercise, chest, front of shoulders and triceps)

(also known as 'Chest Press')

Lay on the bench as before begin with the dumbbells out to the side of the chest, or with a barbell held just above the chest. Slowly extend the arms to their full extent, pause 1-2 seconds at the top of the movement, then lower.

⇨ *Machine equivalent: 'Chest Press Station'*

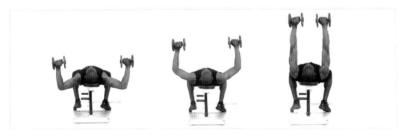

3. Single Arm Dumbbell Rows (back exercise, lats, rear of shoulder and biceps)

Holding the dumbbell at arm's length, rest the other hand and knee on the bench. Slowly raise the arm so the elbow goes as high as possible, then lower to start position. Resist the temptation to "speed up". Some people give the impression they are sawing timber – avoid this at all costs.

⇨ *Machine equivalent: Lat Pull Down Station*

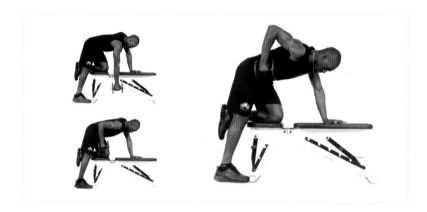

4. Upright Rows (upper back and rear of shoulders exercise)

Stand with feet shoulder width apart holding the barbell or a pair of dumbbells in front of your thighs. The gap between your hands should be about a hands-width. Raise the weights until they are just below the chin (keep your head back to prevent loosening several teeth). Ensure the elbows are raised higher than the shoulders. Pause at the top of the movement for 1-2 seconds then lower to start position.

⇨ *Machine Equivalent: Upright Rows on Cable station using straight bar attachment*

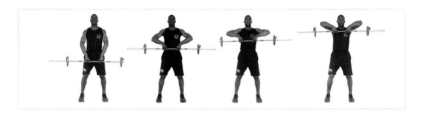

5. Front Raise (shoulder exercise, front of shoulders)

Stand with feet shoulder-width apart with dumbbells resting on each thigh, using an overhand grip. Slowly lift the dumbbells one at a time to shoulder level. Do not raise the second dumbbell until the first dumbbell has returned to the start position. This can also be performed by substituting a barbell and lifting it in the same fashion.

⇨ *Machine Equivalent: cable station*

Not exactly performed the same way, but using the cable station on a low pulley setting allows the same movement. However, you are restricted to performing alternate sets with each arm separately, as opposed to the above which uses alternate arms. This exercise is, however, equally beneficial.

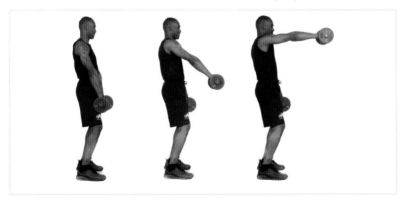

6. Dumbbell Shoulder Press (shoulder exercise, middle and front of shoulders)

Can be performed standing or seated. I prefer the seated version, as I feel it makes it more concentrated. Hold the dumbbells just above the shoulders then extend each arm alternately to the full extent of the arm, rotating the wrist just prior to the completion of the movement so that the hand faces inward. Pause 1-2 seconds, then lower to start position. Alternative versions are to raise both arms simultaneously or use a barbell.

⇨ *Machine Equivalent: Shoulder Press Station*

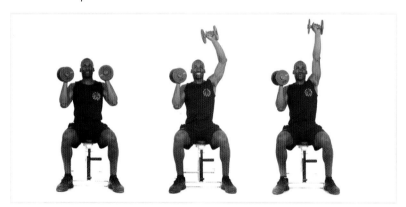

7. Seated bent-over lateral raise (all shoulder area)

While seated, bend forward but maintain a straight back. Hold the dumbbells alongside the ankles, with a slight bend in the arms. Slowly raise the arms out to the side, pause 1-2 seconds, then lower to start position. This exercise can also be performed standing in a bent-over position.

⇨ *Machine Equivalent: Low Pulley Bent-Over Lateral Raises*

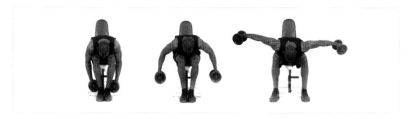

8. Barbell or Dumbbell Squats

(Quads and gluteals. Crudely put – thighs and backside.)

Stand with feet shoulder-width apart with a dumbbell in each hand, held in an overhand grip or with a barbell across the broad part of the rear shoulders (as shown). Look ahead, to ensure a flat back, as you bend the knees until the upper leg is parallel to the floor. Pause 1-2 seconds then return to start position.

⇨ *Machine Equivalent: Leg Press Machine or Squats using 'Smith Machine'*

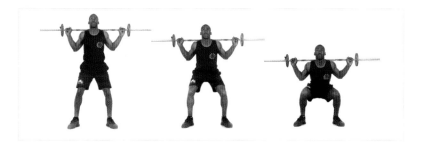

9. Deadlift

(Works just about every muscle you have, but especially all the leg and spinal muscles.)

Correct technique is essential when performing a deadlift. The exercise described here differs from the alternative, the 'Stiff-Legged Deadlift', which is an advanced lift, only for those with a very strong back.

Stand in front of a barbell in such a way that when looking down you can 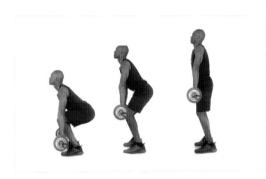 just see the very front tip of your shoes. Maintain a straight back by looking ahead, never down, then bend the knees and grip the bar with an overhand grip, or with a one over, one under grip, if this feels more secure (only experimenting will tell). Slowly lift the bar until it is in front of your thighs – do not bend the arms, keep them straight. Ensure the shoulders are drawn back powerfully at the top of the lift. Pause 2 seconds then lower to within an inch of the floor. Continue in this fashion. If this is too demanding, or you are moving on to heavier weights, you can rest the weight back on the floor between lifts. It is possible to perform the deadlift by using two dumbbells, but I feel using a bar is more effective.

⇨ *Machine Equivalent: Deadlift on the 'Smith Machine'*

10. Dumbbell Bicep Curls (biceps)

There are many variations on the same theme, but I have gone for the basic dumbbell curl, with both weights raised simultaneously. If you find this difficult then lift the dumbbells alternately.

Sit (or stand) with the dumbbells hanging down by your sides then slowly raise them by bending the elbow towards the shoulder. Pause 1-2 seconds then lower to start position.

⇨ *Machine Equivalent: bicep curls on Curl Station or on cable station*

(ideally using E-Z curl bar, which rotates and is shaped especially for this exercise.)

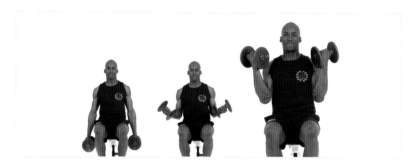

11. Single Arm Seated Triceps Extensions (triceps)

Sit (or stand) holding a dumbbell (a light one if this is the first time you have attempted this exercise) at arm's length above your head. Reach across with the other arm and hold the tricep, this should stabilise the lower arm during the movement to follow. Slowly lower the arm at the elbow out and behind you, finishing behind your neck. My top tip here, which is less obvious than it may seem, is to avoid bringing the weight down on top of your head – I've actually seen it done. Pause 1-2 seconds then return the arm to the starting position.

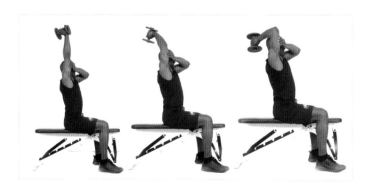

⇨ *Machine Equivalent: Triceps Press-Down Station or Pushdowns on the cable station, using straight bar attachment*

I make no excuses for repeatedly reinforcing the word "slowly" and remembering to "pause"; this should ensure control, safety, sound technique and good results.

12. Barbell Clean and Press (legs, back and shoulders)

Combine working the upper and lower body in the same exercise with this classic lift. Start by standing behind a barbell, ideally an Olympic barbell, with feet shoulder-width apart. Just the tips of your toes should be visible from above, and shins should be close to the bar. Bend the knees to start the lift, hands taking a grip slightly wider than the shoulders, and keeping the head up, with the eyes looking forward to maintain a safe back position; performing this exercise in front of a full-length mirror is very helpful. Lift the bar in one fluid movement to shoulder-height, flipping the palms of the hands over backwards in order to support the bar, which should rest on the upper chest prior to the upward overhead press, in which the arms should be fully extended. Reverse the procedure to lower the bar back to the chest, then, flipping the hands forwards, lower the bar to the floor. Start with an unloaded bar as a rehearsal; in the first few sessions attempt only a few repetitions, adding more as you grow accustomed to the exercise.

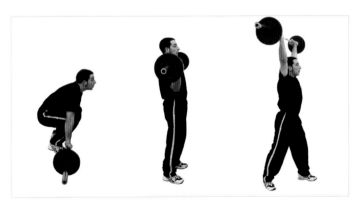

Kettlebells

Although favoured by Russia's special forces, kettlebells were something I initially viewed with some scepticism. I have now come to admit they can play an important part in strength and conditioning training. I particularly like them for deadlifts and squats; I would, however, advise anybody tempted to try them to first get advice from a qualified instructor on safe and proper technique – you would not want one of these articles landing on your foot.

~Tip~
For all-round fitness, don't just depend on weight training. Always try to combine it with cardiovascular training, core training and flexibility training.

Squats

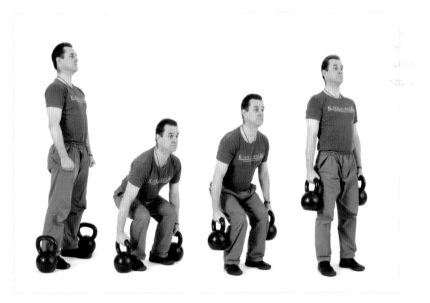

Deadlifts

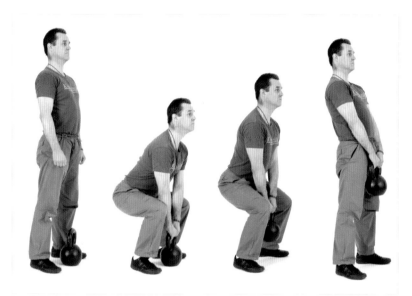

Split routines

If you want to train a little harder, and more often, you may have to split your training up. Performing an all-body workout is the ideal starting procedure, but after a while you may feel the need to intensify your training, and you cannot, as your all-body routine always needs a day off for recovery. It should never be performed on consecutive days. The answer is to split your training into different routines, whereby some of your muscles get a rest, while others are working. You need to work out which muscles to train on which days, so that the same muscles do not get worked on consecutive days. There is a substantial amount of reading matter on this subject, both in books and the great many weight training and bodybuilding magazines available. Always try to get hold of up-to-date literature as some of the older books and periodicals give well-intentioned advice which is now outdated. (See Recommended Reading, opposite.) Below is a basic two day Split Training Routine.

Day 1 and 3

- » Dumbbell Flyes

- » Bench Press

- » Lat pull Downs/ Single arm Rows

- » Bicep Curl

- » Triceps Pressdowns/ Dumbbell Triceps Extensions

- » Abdominals (crunches)

Day 2 and 4

- » Squats

- » Deadlifts

- » Shoulder press

- » Front raise

- » Bent-over lateral raises

- » Upright rows

- » Abdominals (reverse curls)

Informed reading or advice from your instructor can help you tailor your own routines.

Recommended Reading

The Complete Guide to Strength Training by Anita Bean (A & C Black)

Strength Training Anatomy by Frederic Delavier.

For advanced trainers:
Brawn and *Beyond Brawn* by Stuart McRobert (Common Sense Publishing)

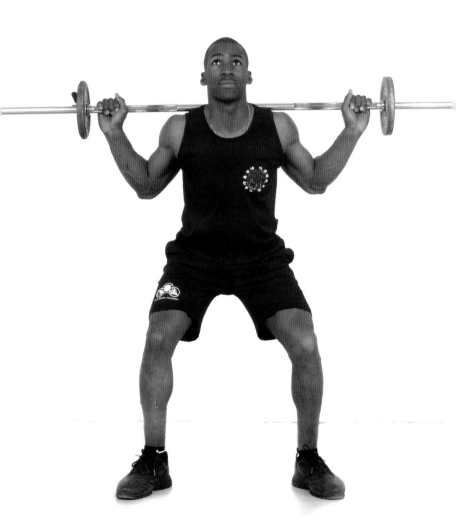

Circuit training at home / at the gym

ALTHOUGH PEOPLE – PARTICULARLY THOSE IN THE MILITARY forces – have worked out in a way that we would recognise as circuit training for many years, apparently the term was coined at the University of Leeds in the late 1950's.[§] You may have done circuit training before, possibly at a gym or as part of training for football, rugby, or any sport which requires a combination of strength and stamina. It usually involves a number of exercise stations set around a hall, gym space or a field. At each, you work out for either the allotted time or number of repetitions, then progress to the next station. Doing it at home will be slightly different (unless you inhabit a cavernous mansion or loft), but for those training in the boxroom, shed, garage or wherever else you have chosen, you will be doing it in the confines of that space – picking up or putting down different exercise apparatus. It is not complicated, or, I assure you, I would not have been teaching it since what seems like the Fall of Rome.

The beauty of circuit training is its flexibility to be adapted to an individual's specific fitness or training demands.

Unless you are doing the class at a fitness centre and somebody is keeping the tempo by barking out instructions, you can feel free to go at your own pace; I would suggest working 30-40 seconds or 10-20 repetitions at each 'station'.

The type of circuit I have provided in this section is intended purely as an example; you can modify it as you feel appropriate to fulfil your personal aims, or simply make your own circuit up, composed of stations you feel best match your needs.

I always try to spread out the pushing and pulling exercises so they never run consecutively; the biceps (used in pulling) and the triceps (used in pushing) are among the smaller muscle groups and need longer to recover. I also space out the leg exercises as I feel it may prove debilitating to perform them

---

[§] According to Manfred Scholich in his in-depth manual "Circuit Training For All Sports," published in 1992 (SBP Books)

consecutively in a circuit, unless a weight-bearing exercise (such as squats) is followed by an aerobic exercise (such as skipping or jogging.) Decide if you want to focus on aerobic fitness, muscular strength or endurance or, as I favour in my examples, a combination of each.

Rest 20-30 seconds between stations, depending on the intensity level of the exercises.

(Fitter people can rest 10-15 seconds, dependent on the intensity of the exercises; the very fit can just carry on regardless without a rest.)

Keep water handy – sip as you go.

The following warm up is crucial, to get your heart rate up and prepare you for the circuit:

Warm-up

5 minutes of jogging in place, skipping or shadow boxing (see 'Boxing Training').

Mobility

The mobilisation stage is important. This is where you need to get some synovial fluid (the juice that oils our joints) into your joints.

- *Neck:* Look over your shoulder, drop your chin to gaze at the ground as you slowly turn to look over the other shoulder

- *Shoulders:* Slowly rotate your arms forward and back a few times

- *Knees:* Support your upper body as you raise the knee to form a right angle behind you. Perform in a slow flowing manner for several repetitions.

- *Ankle:* Slowly rotate your ankle in circles three or four times clockwise and then anti-clockwise. Point the toe then bring the toe up toward the shin in an up and down motion.

- *Wrists:* Slowly rotate your wrist in circles and follow by shaking the fingers as if flicking water off them.

Short stretch: see section on the One Minute Stretch, page 151.

Exercises

1. Press-ups

If you are not yet up to full press-ups, get yourself started with "box" press-ups (hands and knees on the floor) as opposed to "full" press-ups (hands and toes on the floor).

Whichever type you are doing, start by placing the hands below the shoulders or slightly wider, whichever seems more natural.

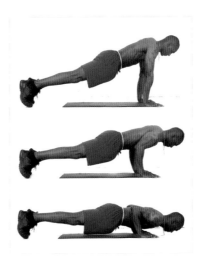

- Start with 10-20 repetitions

- Progress to 25 press-ups, or 30 seconds continuous.

- Make 50 full press-ups (performed correctly) your goal.

2. Step-ups

(Use the stairs, doorstep or a sturdy crate.)

As you step, the leg you step up with should form a right angle.

- 10 step-ups each leg

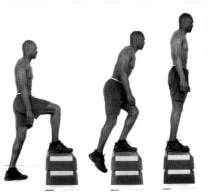

- Progress to 20 step-ups each leg

- Progress to the above while holding dumbbells.

3. Back extensions

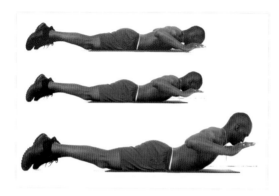

Lie face down on a mat, and, keeping hips on the floor, slowly raise the upper body. Bend elbows out to the side so your fingers are barely touching your ears.

• Start with 15 reps

• Progress to 30 seconds continuous.

4. Shadow box (see boxing training)

- Start with 1 minute round

- Progress to 2/3 minute rounds.

5. Curls – abdominals

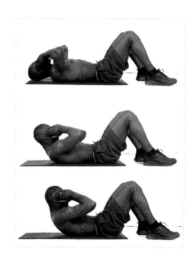

Lie on a mat with your knees bent at right angles. Bend your elbows so your fingers rest lightly against the side of your head – do not pull on your head since this will give you neck pain from hell! Slowly raise your head until your shoulder blades (not your back) are off the floor. Pause for two seconds, then lower.

- Start with 15-20 curl-ups

- Progress to 30-50.

Progress to "crunches" where the legs are raised off the floor at a right angle; raise the head towards the knees, ensuring lower back stays on the floor.

- Start with 15-20 crunches

- Progress to 30-50.

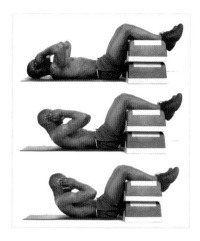

6. Stick hops (any stick will do!)

Place 4-6 sticks (each about 2 feet/ 60cm in length) on the floor, around 2 feet/60cm apart. Take two-footed hops to land between the sticks both forwards and sideways.

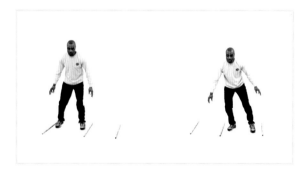

- Start with 20 hops

- Progress to 30-60 seconds continuous.

7. Calf raises

Stand on a step box or sturdy crate, or, if at home, the bottom stair, with your heels hanging over the edge behind you, while you are supported by your hands against the wall or handrail. Slowly go up on your toes, and then allow your heels to drop below the level of the box/stair.

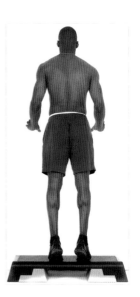

- 20 reps

- Progress to 30 seconds

- Progress to 20-30 seconds while holding a dumbbell in one hand.

8. Triceps dips

Grip the edge of a bench, hands palm down behind you. Slowly lower your body by bending the arms, then return to start position.

- 20 repetitions

- Progress to 30-60 seconds continuous

- Progress to the above with feet elevated on another chair/box.

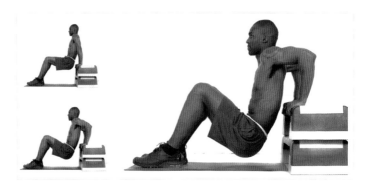

9. Squats

Stand with feet shoulder width apart. Looking straight ahead, hold your arms out to the front, for balance. Bend your knees until your thighs are parallel to the floor. Hold for 1-2 seconds then return slowly to the start position.

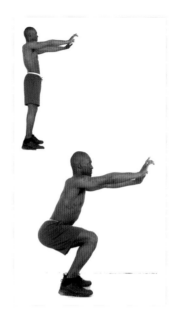

- Start with 20 repetitions

- Progress to 20 repetitions holding dumbbells in each hand. Do not bend the arm at any time during the exercise; the arm stays straight down by your side.

Gradually increase a) the weight of the dumbbells if you want to improve strength or b) the number of repetitions, if you want to increase endurance.

10. Reverse curls

Lie on your back on a mat. Raise your legs, crossed at the ankles for stability, into a right angle. Slowly draw your knees towards your upper body until your backside, not your lower back, is off the floor. Slowly return to the start position.

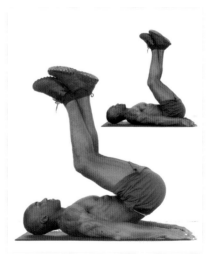

- 10-20 repetitions

- Progress to 30 seconds continuous.

11. Lunges

Start by standing with feet shoulder width apart. Step forward with one leg until both the front and back leg form right angles. Place the hands on the hips or out to the side (like a tightrope walker); experiment to discover whichever you find suits you best for balance.

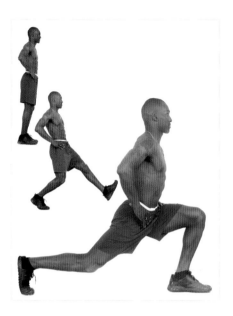

- Alternate leg lunges 30 seconds continuous

- Progress to 30-60 seconds while holding a dumbbell in each hand.

12. Squat thrusts/burpees

Squat with your hands on the floor in front of you. Supported by your hands, thrust your legs back to their full length with what will be, hopefully, a dynamic action. Immediately return your knees to your arms to complete a "squat thrust".

- As above but stand up rapidly at the completion of each squat thrust before

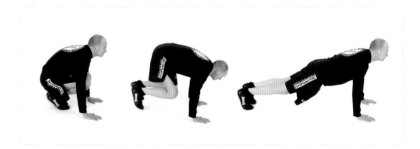

dropping back to the original position. This stand-up insertion serves to make the exercise that little bit harder.

- 20 squat thrusts

- Progress to 30 seconds

- Progress to 20 burpees

- Progress to 30-60 seconds of burpees.

13. Plank

(also referred to as "Hovers" and "The Bridge")

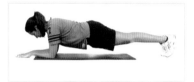

Lie face down on a mat supported by your elbows and toes. Your arms should be bent at right angles, the elbows directly below the shoulders. Use a mirror or ask a friend to check your body is parallel to the floor; try not to sag or stick your backside up in the air.

Contract your abdominal muscles but do not hold your breath; breathe normally. A superb exercise for ratcheting up your mid-section.

- Hold the position for 30-60 seconds

- Progress to holding for 2 minutes or longer.

14. Side plank

The sideway version of the above, and just slightly more challenging.

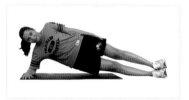

Facing sideways, support yourself on one elbow and one foot, with your legs together, and your body straight. Work alternate sides.

This is a great exercise for the obliques, so even though you may be grimacing, content yourself with the thought that your love-handles are disappearing.

- Hold for 30 seconds each side

- Progress to 1-2 minutes or longer on each side.

15. Skipping

- Skip for two minutes.

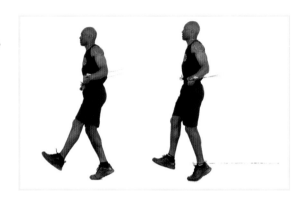

16. Tuck jumps

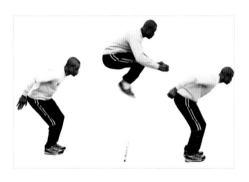

Start with feet shoulder-width apart. Half squat before making a vertical take-off, bringing the knees up towards the chest. Land softly with bent knees to absorb the shock. Take a few light bounces prior to "taking off" again.

- Start with a 30 second session

- Progress to 1-2 minutes.

17. Standing twists

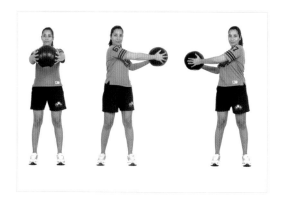

Stand with a medicine ball held in extended, but relaxed, arms, out in front of you. Turn to the side as if about to give the ball to somebody behind you. Come back to the centre and pause 1-2 seconds before making the same manoeuvre to the other side.

* Start with 20 repetitions

* Progress to 30-60 repetitions.

18. Chins

Challenging but rewarding is how I can best describe this exercise. Grasp an overhead bar with a wide overhand grip (or a narrow underhand grip to start with) then pull yourself up until your chin is bar high – in other words, until you have "chinned" it. Great for the back and shoulders, but it is in the arms you will feel it most.

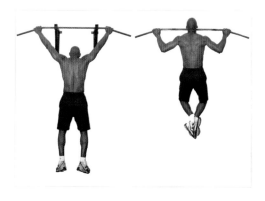

- Start by going for your personal best

- Try to add 1-2 repetitions each time you perform the exercise.

Cooldown/warmdown: 5 minutes

Relaxed skipping, shadow boxing, or jogging (on the spot if space is limited).

Cooldown/warmdown stretch

A long stretch (20-30 seconds per body part). See Stretching, page 143.

Moving on

To move on from this stage you can gradually incorporate some home-friendly equipment. "Home-friendly" means the kit can live in the garage, shed, loft or even the cupboard under the stairs if you can squeeze it in.

Swiss ball, fitball, exercise ball (whatever)

A fit-ball, Swiss Ball, Exercise Ball, Physio Ball, Stability Ball or whatever you want to call it (it's just 'the big ball' at our gym) is of great benefit for both versatility, fitness and balance improvement. For an in-depth look at training with this apparatus, see the section on "Swiss ball training", from which you can add additional exercises to your circuit training.

Skipping rope

Skipping can be done at whatever pace you like – you will still derive some benefit from it. Ropes are cheap (I've seen them for as little as £2.99), but spending about £10 will get you a top quality specimen. For all you ever needed to know about skipping and skipping ropes – see Skipping, page 54.

Tubi-grip/ exercise tubing

Tubi-grip (also referred to as Exertube) is another useful addition, allowing you to do resistance training without using weights; it is versatile and reasonably inexpensive. It is colour-coded to reveal the degree of difficulty of use, black being the most resistant. Green tubigrip is ideal for those at Level 1. Reebok market a variety that is adjustable in length and comes in four varying strength levels.

Dynabands/exercise bands

These stretchy latex strips, usually three feet by six inches in size (but can be bought by the roll and cut to required length) are a simple yet effective training method, allowing the user to perform a wide range of pushing and pulling exercises. The main problem as I see it is that there is no universal colour code; suppliers use their own colours for differing strengths, which can be confusing. Dynabands is a trade name, but one which I, and most fitness instructors in the UK, would recognise. It uses a colour code as follows:

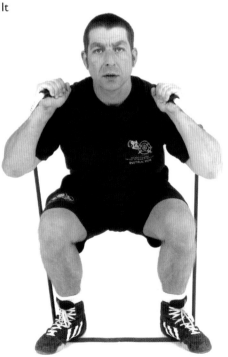

» Beginner = pink

» Intermediate = green

» Advanced = black

Training at home with Dynabands can be combined with other items, such as the fit-ball, or just wrapped around a stair post to give an improvised pushing or pulling station.

Weights

A set of different weights will be of great value for home circuit training, as you will benefit from variety. The weights you perform squats with will, ideally, be a little heavier than those you do lateral raise or bicep curls with, but only buy what you need, especially if you are only going to use them once or twice a week.

Stepbox

Reebok and similar makers market a purpose-built step box, but if you are price conscious (they cost £34 at the time of writing) get hold of a sturdy milk/bread/packing crate or use your, or a friend's, woodworking skills to assemble your own box.

Place a rubber mat underneath it for added stability. A box, for doing step-ups, calf raises or similar exercises, is extremely handy.

Punchbag

Discussed in detail in "boxing training", a punch bag is the greatest stress reliever I know of. Berating a punch bag for a few minutes results in a feeling of tension and anxiety ebbing from you – as good as an analyst and much cheaper, since punchbags range from about £30 (vinyl/PVC) for makes such as BBE, Blitz or Tornado, all of whom do a good line in affordable boxing equipment. A high-end leather bag by Reyes or Everlast will take you into the three figure bracket, but you get pretty much what you pay for in this market.

Utility weights bench

A purpose built bench can be bought new for around £60. The Reebok bench at Argos can be used in a flat position for such exercises as 'bench press', or as a seating unit for exercises such as 'seated shoulder press'. Benches can be quite easily picked up second-hand, and even a solid bench with a worn or tatty-looking cover can be re-covered quite simply and cheaply.

The Reebok deck

I feel it is worth making a brief mention of this piece of equipment as I have used one, (there is one at the gym where I work, but I would gladly have one at home), and was quite pleased with its capability. It can be used as a step-box, or a higher platform box; a weight training bench (as long as you are not incredibly tall or over 20 stone); it also can be used as an incline bench and a decline bench. It has a compartment for rubber exercise tubes which can be slotted into recesses in the bench to enable them to be used for resistance.

Exercise mats

Vital! You absolutely need one of these, even if you have a luxurious carpet in the lounge or bedroom, you should still get a mat, in order to train comfortably anywhere you like. No need to pay the earth: Argos sell a Pro Fitness model for £3.99, or a Reebok mat for £6.99. I have seen versions that sell for £1.99. On a personal note, I lashed out £9.99 for a Gold's Gym version (from J.J.B Sports), with which I am extremely satisfied (not always the case with some stuff I've dragged home). It is a good size, can be wiped down, and has thick padding – handy for those with any sort of back problem.

Press-up stands

Currently on sale for about a fiver in Argos, these are a great piece of transportable equipment to assist your press-ups by allowing more range and taking pressure away from the wrists. Ideal for training at home as they take up hardly any space and can be used on any surface.

Core training on the Swiss ball

CORE TRAINING MEANS TRAINING THE MUSCLES OF THE torso which provide stability. It has become commonplace in most gyms now, and although in years gone by Swiss ball training was unheard of, most people were doing some kind of core training – for instance, press-ups and crunches – as part of their fitness routine. The introduction of the Swiss ball gave a new dimension to this kind of training. Admittedly, I sneered at it originally, but I have come to use it in training with an increased frequency over the years.

This item of equipment goes by various names: the Fitball, Stability Ball, Mediball, Physio Ball and the Gym-ball are just some other variations I have heard, but it was first introduced as the Swiss ball, so I'm sticking with that.

It was first introduced by Swiss remedial therapists to assist primarily with back problems, and at best was treated with curiosity, and oft-times with derision, on its earliest ingress to gymnasiums. It has nevertheless grown in popularity due to the variety of exercises it allows. You use numerous muscles merely to stop yourself falling off the thing.

The extra effort required to manage the additional element of instability allows for core improvements both in strength and balance. The idea is that the unstable surface will place additional challenges to the trunk muscles in order to provide improved spinal balance and stability. It takes a little getting used to at first and I would suggest using it on a soft surface to begin with – just in case.

Know your limits

Do not try any complicated exercises until you feel completely confident laying backward on the ball. In many gyms the Swiss ball has been used as a substitute for the weights bench; this is all well and good, provided the weights are not heavy – if they are it is far better, and safer, to use a bench. (I've never seen anyone fall off a bench with weights in their hands, but I've heard cases of this happening on Swiss balls when excessive weight was used.) I have never yet heard of a bench bursting or being punctured – however, rarely, this may happen to a Swiss ball. (It is usually when some imbecile has left a sharp object lying about on the floor.)I also strongly advise against standing on the Swiss ball; kneeling on the ball in a safe environment i.e. on a judo mat, is an aid to improving balance, but standing on the ball carries, in my view, no benefit that is worth the high likelihood of an accident.

Make sure your ball is always fully inflated (the cheaper, thinner-skinned models seem to go down more quickly) and keep it well away from sharp edges of gym equipment, tools and furniture.

Get the size right first

The following is a general guide used by most Swiss ball retailers, and I have found it to be fairly reliable:

User's Height	Ball Size
4' 8" – 5' 5" (140 – 160cm)	55 cm
5' 6" – 6' 0" (165 – 185cm)	65cm
6' plus	75cm

Most manufacturers state that the maximum load is 300kg, but, although I'd advise against putting this to a practical test, I do know of a 30 stone giant of a man who uses his as an office chair.

There are numerous books (see list at end of section), videos and DVD's dedicated to Swiss ball exercises, but in the following section I have provided a basic workout.

I have added a medicine ball in some of the exercises but they can be performed without a ball, or with a dumbbell.

Exercises

1. Wall Squat

Place the ball between a wall and your back. Looking ahead and keeping your

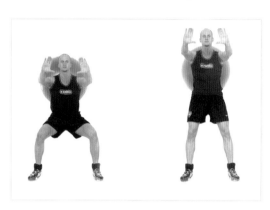

body straight, bend into a squat position until your thighs are parallel with the floor. Hold for 1-2 seconds then return to start position. Keep the pressure on the ball by constantly leaning back into it in order to retain it as it rolls up and down with you.

2. Press-ups

There are two different press-up techniques which can be employed; both are, in my experience, challenging.

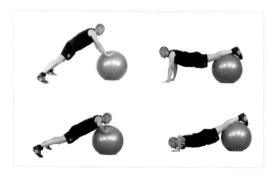

• Rest your hands firmly on the ball, ensure your body is straight (check in the mirror or ask somebody). Lower your chest down onto the ball, pause 1-2 seconds and return to start position. The slower you work the more control you should have.

- Place your insteps on the ball and, ensuring your body is straight, lower yourself to the floor, pause 1-2 seconds and then return to the start position. To make it harder try to do this with the tips of your toes on the ball.

3. Curls

Begin by sitting on the ball. Slowly walk your feet forward, allowing your lower back to come to a rest on the ball. With just the tips of your fingers touching your head, progress to now curling your body upward, then slowly coming down again. Pause for 1-2 seconds at the top and bottom of the exercise. To make this a little more demanding you can hold a medicine ball.

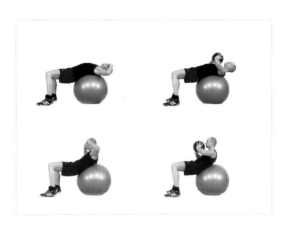

4. Back Extensions

Lie on the ball resting on your mid-section. With your elbows out to the sides (as if giving a double salute) slowly lift your upper body, pause for 1-2 seconds, then lower to the start position.

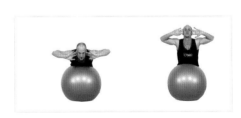

5. Russian Twists

Lay on your back on the ball in the same start position as curls (no.3). Fully extend your arms above you. If you do not have a medicine ball, football or dumbbell simply place the palms of the hands together. Roll

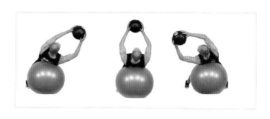

to alternate sides, coming to rest on the shoulder at the completion of the turn.

6. Jack Knife

These are also referred to as 'reverse roll-ins'; start as if about to do a press-up with the legs on the ball (see 2). Bend your knees to roll the ball toward you. Pause 1-2

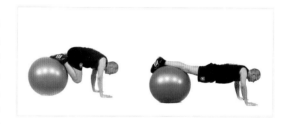

seconds then roll the ball back by extending your legs.

7. Lateral Curls

Lay sideways on the ball with the elbows out to the side giving a double salute. If this is difficult at first, try holding onto the ball with the lower arm, instead of bending the elbow. It may also help to start

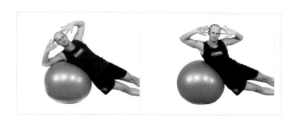

with your feet against the base of a wall. Once you are in position raise your upper body sideways as far as you can, pause for 1-2 seconds, then return to the start position.

8. Plank

Rest your hands on the Swiss ball in the same position as you would to perform a press-up. Contract your abdominal muscles but don't hold your breath as you maintain a stable position for as long as you can.

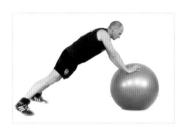

9. Kneeling on the Ball

The ultimate balance test. Make sure you are next to a wall or a stable surface (I prefer a stack of judo mats). Start with the ball on a judo mat or a large gym mat if this is possible – please do not attempt this where there is a concrete floor! Climb onto the ball with both hands and one leg, then hoist the other leg onto the ball, holding on to the wall for support if you feel unstable. Try to let go of your support as you come up into a kneeling position with your arms outstretched for balance, akin to a tightrope walker. Use a timer to see how long you can last, always striving to beat your previous best. Never stand on the ball: the danger outweighs any benefit.

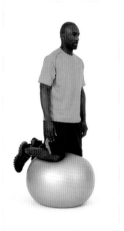

Recommended reading

Lisa Westlake *Strong to the Core* (Arum Press) & *Get on the Ball* (Apple Press)

Lorne Goldenberg and Peter Twist *Strength Ball Training* (Human Kinetics)

Matt Lawrence *Core Stability* (A & C Black)

The boxing workout

Why Boxing Training?

It improves strength, speed, co-ordination, aerobic and anaerobic fitness, agility, muscular and cardiovascular endurance.

If you are suffering from feelings of frustration, depression or anger, I can assure you that bashing a punch bag will give you a refreshing sense of release, and make you feel a whole lot better.

A company director I had trained returned to buy a punch bag and gloves for his sales staff, to allow them to batter it when they became frustrated with their job.

The where and the when

If you do not have any home space for this workout you need to seek out an appropriate gym. It may be one of those new, air-conditioned, shiny gyms with racks of equipment, but it may well be a converted church hall, with a wooden floor and fluorescent lighting; it may well be more gritty than glamorous, but if it is friendly and has punch bags and some decent space, don't be afraid to try it. Even the new gyms have realised that there is more to boxing fitness than they previously considered and have installed punch bags and employed instructors who will teach people to skip rope and hold focus pads which teach people how to box. You need somewhere, ideally, that has access to a punch bag and space to skip and do your shuttle runs; many gyms have a quiet time between the lunchtime and evening class (I know our gym does) where you can take advantage of such facilities to work alone.

Equipment

It is possible that the gym is where you will find your punch

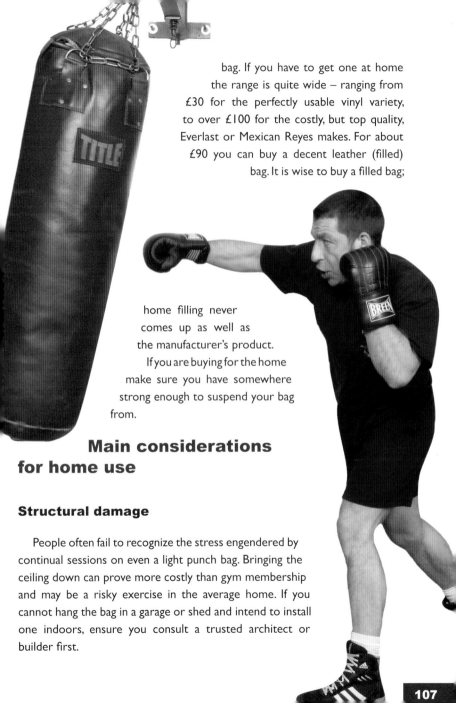

bag. If you have to get one at home the range is quite wide – ranging from £30 for the perfectly usable vinyl variety, to over £100 for the costly, but top quality, Everlast or Mexican Reyes makes. For about £90 you can buy a decent leather (filled) bag. It is wise to buy a filled bag; home filling never comes up as well as the manufacturer's product. If you are buying for the home make sure you have somewhere strong enough to suspend your bag from.

Main considerations for home use

Structural damage

People often fail to recognize the stress engendered by continual sessions on even a light punch bag. Bringing the ceiling down can prove more costly than gym membership and may be a risky exercise in the average home. If you cannot hang the bag in a garage or shed and intend to install one indoors, ensure you consult a trusted architect or builder first.

Noise

Your neighbours, or even your nearest and dearest, are likely to suffer if there is a constant tattoo and sound of dull thuds rendered by your efforts.

Fittings and Fixings

These can work out costly if you have to employ somebody to install your bag, and unless space is not at a premium you may have a storage problem. Those sharing your home may not view a punch bag as a particularly attractive feature if it is constantly on view.

A free-standing bag can cost from £120-£250, which, unlike a wall-hung bag, allows for 360 degree movement. The downside is the weight of free-standing bags; to stabilise them they need the base to be filled with sand or water, so it is advisable to ensure your floor is strong enough to take it.

If hanging the bag on a wall bracket, first take advice on the strength of the bricks. "Soft" bricks will come away from the wall with the bracket still attached (I've witnessed this twice), so seek a builder's advice first.

There are different variations of punch bags. If your gym has a teardrop bag, an uppercut bag or similar then why not try them out. If you are a newcomer and the heavy bag is a little unforgiving, try starting on something less demanding.

Hands and gloves

I always advise getting your own punch bag mitts, unless you have fragile hands, in which case you should wear sparring gloves, which are larger and more heavily padded to protect your hands.

Some gyms have a "lucky dip" box in which gloves unloved and abandoned by their owners now sadly reside. This may seem a reasonable idea, but unfortunately it has seemed that way to many other people before you came along, and if you are unlucky you can finish up with hands bearing the fragrance of performing seals, which no cleanser known to mankind can dispel - for at least a day or two. Given they may be ill-fitting into the bargain, I strongly advise you to take the plunge and buy your own punch-bag mitts. I've seen them for as little as £10.

As stated above I always advise people to get their own gloves, and to always buy good quality leather ones. The vinyl type tend to wear out quickly, offer less protection and are prone to splitting.

Ensure you have a little room left in your gloves, for two reasons,

» Your hands will become hot if you wear the gloves for a long session and they will swell slightly

» You would be well advised to wrap your hands, especially if you intend to work on the heavy bag; leave adequate space for the wraps.

Hand Wraps

You can provide further protection for your hands by using wraps. There are ready-made versions which you can wear inside your mitts, but I prefer the wraps you apply in bandage form as they can be moulded into a perfect fit.

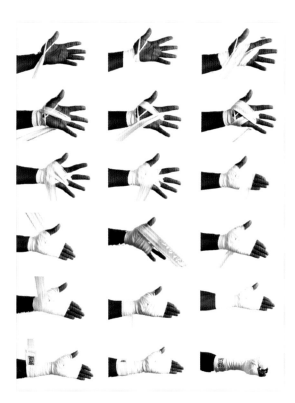

Footwear

As the workout involves skipping and shuttle runs I would advise wearing running shoes.

Technique

How to hit the bag, and how to shadow box, require a detailed explanation for you to get the most out of this workout. The information I give here is for right-handed people, setting up with the left foot forward. If you are left-handed, my apologies – simply reverse all right and left-handed instructions. Everything is the same, just the other way round.

Hitting the bag

Making a fist suitable for the job may seem obvious but I still find newcomers who are unsure where to place the thumb. Most injuries that beginners sustain are to the wrist (through failure to keep a straight arm on contact), or to the thumb (due to incorrect placement of the thumb). With this in mind;

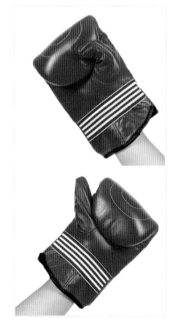

- settle the hand comfortably in the glove, pulling hard on the wristband to ensure a snug (but not tight) fit. When buying gloves try them on wearing hand-wraps if you intend to use them.

- close the fingers of the hand leaving the thumb in the "thumbs up" position.

- draw the thumb tightly down against the fingers; the thumb MUST be retained in this position to guard against injury.

The Stance

Imagine you are standing on a clock face, your left foot on 12 o'clock and your right foot at twenty past twelve. Try to stay close to this stance, never cross your feet.

Your bodyweight leans minimally forward from the waist. You are not bolt upright but slightly crouched. Your chin is low enough to have a tennis ball trapped underneath it, but your eyes should

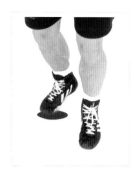

be on the target. Both elbows are tucked comfortably against the ribs and the right hand is close to the chin. The left hand is held at the same height as the right, but about a foot ahead of it. Arms and legs should feel relaxed: loose limbs travel faster and smoother, so avoid tension at all costs.

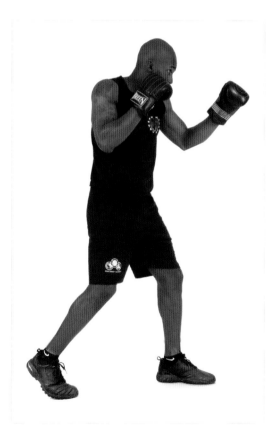

Movement

All you need to remember when you first start is this simplified guide to direct your movements;

a)   the front foot takes you forward

b)   the back foot takes you backward

c)   to go to the right, push off with the left foot

d)   to go to the left, push off with the right foot

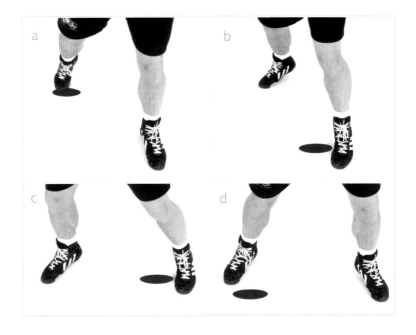

Step and Slide

Stay on the balls of your feet and practice maintaining good balance as you move around. Do not bounce (this just wastes energy); move in a sliding fashion.

As you step forward with the front foot, allow the rear foot to slide in the same direction. Try to glide like a ballroom dancer – a tough ballroom dancer.

The Punches

For purposes of these exercises we will be using 3 punches:

- the jab

- the straight right (or right cross)

- the hook.

The left jab

This is quite a natural action, delivered sharply and cleanly, more like a spear than a club. Just snap the left glove to the target in a straight line, landing with

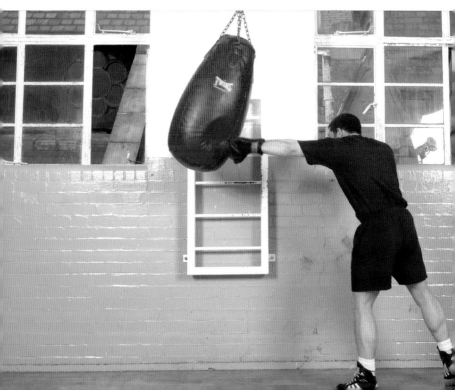

the knuckle part of the glove. Turn the left hip and shoulder as you do for a little added power. The most important part of throwing a punch is the transfer of weight. When you jab you should use the ball of the right (rear) foot to propel your weight forward, stepping a few inches forward with the left (front) foot; try to picture somebody standing on the toes of your right (rear) foot as you get the 'feel'. Don't let the back foot come off the ground – try to avoid an 'Eros' look as you finish.

Directly after making contact retract the glove to the basic stance position.

The Straight Right/Right Cross

This is where you can turn the power on, which is why the 'big' hand stays back instead of leading. This is hitting off your naturally stronger wing, and brings the full satisfying feeling that accompanies it as you zing it into the bag. This is not a spear – this is a trip-hammer. As with the jab you will need the transference of weight, driving off the ball of the right foot, turning the hip and shoulder in the direction of the target. The upper row of knuckles are the hardest part of the hand, so attempt to punch slightly downwards on impact to ensure this part of the hand makes contact first. Stay upright, keeping the shoulders over the hips, to avoid 'reaching' for the target in such a way that the upper body leans forward, which will result in a large loss of power.

When you go forward – take your hips with you, don't let the shoulders get ahead of the hips. Try not to list over to your left (which is a common error). The left side of your body should allow the right side to pivot, as it acts like a hinge. Do not drop the left hand as you throw the right, keep it alongside your face. Keep chin down and eyes on the target and retract the right glove, along the same line as it went out, directly after contact.

The Hook

The left hand comes back to the action now, with a classic, short, hard punch. To launch the hook, shift your weight to the side you intend to strike from, the left in this case, turning the hip and shoulder slightly away from the target. Your arm is bent at the elbow, at about 90 degrees. The other hand is kept close to the head. By rapidly raising the heel and pivoting the hip of the hitting

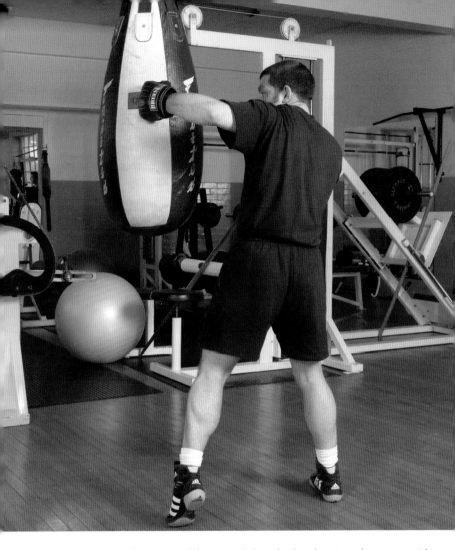

side simultaneously, make a powerful turn and slam the hand against the target with the upper knuckles leading, and the thumb (tucked in tightly) on top at contact. The instant after hitting, whip the hand back to the start position, so you could repeat the punch if you wanted to. If you have trouble turning your hips bring the rear foot forward a few inches.

For a right hook simply peel away to your right and then take the same action as you did with the left.

Variations on a Hooking Theme

The shape of the hitting arm will dictate the amount of power applied when throwing the hook.

*   if the arm is bent at the elbow to form a right angle this will encourage a strong hip turn which will result in greater punching power

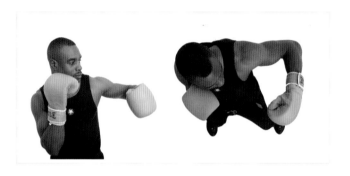

*   if the arm is at an 'obtuse angle' – greater than a right angle – there will be reduced power as there is less hip turn

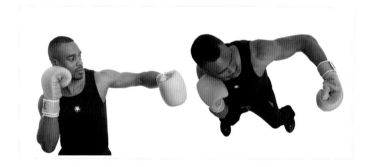

- when the arm forms an 'acute angle', with the fist closer to the body, a full forceful hip turns needs to be applied to register a punch with the arm in this form, resulting in an extremely strong impact from very close range.

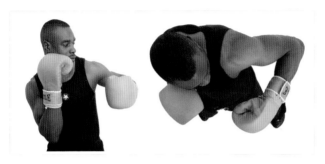

TIP: for all varieties of the hook try bringing the rear foot slightly forward to a 'quarter past twelve' position.

Shadow Boxing

This is a good exercise on its own, and gives you the chance to get used to the footwork, and throw all the punches. Only throw punches at your imaginary target when you stop moving – leave hitting on the move to legends like Ali. Don't put too much effort or power into your punches. Stay totally relaxed throughout. Don't extend the arms fully or lock your elbows out. Try to keep in the '20 past 12' position as you cruise around. There is no need to wear your gloves as (hopefully) you won't be hitting anything. If you can find a partner to work opposite you, this will give a realistic sense

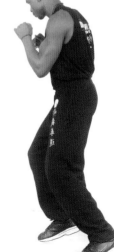

of purpose to your efforts – but keep enough distance between you and your partner, about 5-6 feet, to prevent accidental and painful knuckle bumping (or worse).

The workout activities

Start with a 5 minute warm-up: skipping, shadow boxing or a combination of both.

Short stretch (see Stretching, page 141) and mobilise joints.

For this exercise it is a good idea to stretch the hand and forearm muscles. This is done to protect the elbow and wrist joints and the associated ligaments against the shock of hitting the bag. Run through these stretches after your workout as well.

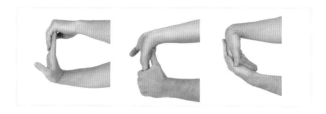

Here are some combinations you can try to give you some variation in your workouts

    a)   Jab, straight right, left hook, right hook.

    b)   Jab, jab, straight right, left hook

    c)   Left hook high, left hook low (waist high), right hook

    d)   Jab low, jab high, straight right, left hook

    e)   Jab, low straight right, left hook, straight right

f)   Jab, left hook, right hook, right hook low.

g)   Jab, jab, right hook, left hook, straight right.

If you are fortunate enough to train at a gym which has a speed-ball, a floor-to-ceiling ball or any other punch bags, try to incorporate them into your workout to add more variety. The above should only be used as a rough guide. Change or substitute exercises as you wish to suit your own taste and needs.

The Solo Workout

Preparation

You don't want to overrun your allotted time so if there is a large/visible clock, that will be handy, as most people prefer to remove their watch when wearing bag mitts. You cannot look at a watch while skipping or punching a bag, so an audible device is ideal. This is where a timer with a countdown facility comes in handy, or an kitchen timer that 'dings' at zero, a stopwatch with an audible alarm, or a Casio G-shock or Timex Ironman with an audible alarm. Usually mobile phones have a countdown timer. The one on my Nokia is suitably loud but the one on my Oregon Scientific heart rate monitor is pitifully quiet making it woefully inadequate. So you need to have one eye on the clock or a device that has an alarm perceptible above the sound of a skipping rope, a bag being walloped or a thumping stereo system.

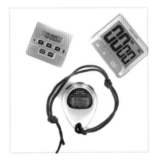

Have some water standing by, in order to sip as you go and a towel if you think you will need it. I'll be surprised, not to mention disappointed, if this little lot doesn't make you sweat.

⇨ *The solo workout: programme*

			1	2	3
1	Skip 2 minutes	2 mins			
2	The one-minute stretch (p. 151)	1 min			
3	Shadow box Throw jabs, straight rights and hooks from both hands as you move around, remembering the 20 past 12 stance with your footwork. This will get your body heat back up after your stretch and act as a rehearsal for the punch bag. Use only half power in your punching.	2 mins			
4	Punch bag – on your first session, hit light and fast	2 mins			
5	Skip, at an easy pace	2 mins			
6	Crunches on the floor or Swiss ball	20 reps			
7	Step-ups (10 on each leg) with or without weights	20 reps			
8	Punch bag: solid hitting. Really get stuck in	2 mins			
9	Squats, with or without weights	20 reps			
10	Skip: fast pace	2 mins			
11	Press ups	20 reps			
12	Shuttle run	2 mins			
13	Punch bag (same as #8)	2 mins			
14	Reverse curls	20 reps			
15	Skip: relaxed pace	3 mins			
16	Walk – hands on hips, take deep inhalations to get your breath back	2 mins			
17	Warm down stretch				

Gym work / homework

ALTHOUGH SPACE AND EQUIPMENT MAY BE MORE ACCESSIBLE at the gym, much of this work can be achieved at home with a minimal amount of equipment. The exercises all require very little room to perform.

Below is a menu of various exercises from which you can select the ones you feel you can fit into your workout. I have only added explanation where I feel the exercise is not obvious.

Several of these exercises are also included in Circuit Training and Core Training, others from those sections can be inserted or substituted here when you want to design your own workout.

The exercises

1. Curl-ups

Lay on your back on a mat with bent knees. Raise upper body to take the shoulder blades off the floor but not the lower back.

    a)   On mat

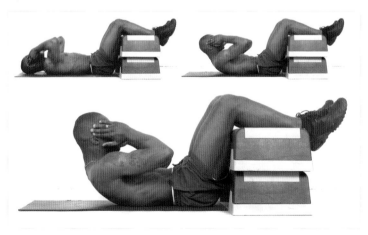

b)   On decline Reebok deck

Laying on a declined deck, curl the upper body forward but leave lower back on the bench.

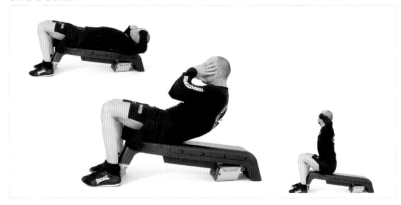

2. Crunches/curl-ups on Swiss ball (see Core Training)

a)   empty hands

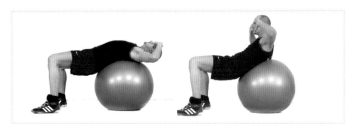

b)   with medicine ball

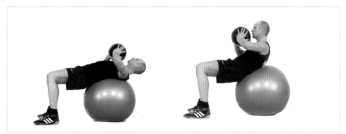

3. Reverse curls with feet elevated (on step-box, deck or bench)

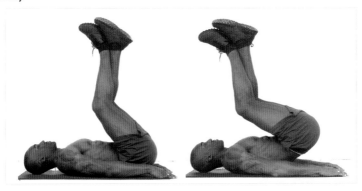

4. Russian Twist on Swiss ball & standing twists

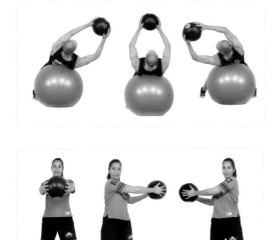

Russian Twists on Swiss ball – see Core Training, page 100.

Standing Twists: stand feet shoulder-width apart, arms full extended in front of you, holding a medicine ball, preferably a two-handled one. Slowly make a full turn to alternate sides.

5. Plank/Bridge

On all the plank exercises, contract the abdominal muscles as if attempting to pull your navel inward.

Do not hold your breath.

a) On elbows
b) On Swiss ball
c) Feet up on Swiss ball

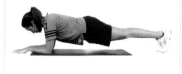

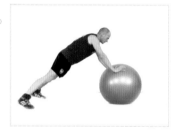

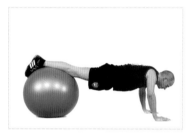

6. Side plank – left & right

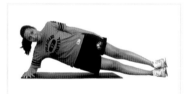

7. Step-ups

Step-ups using weights or medicine ball (as depicted but holding a dumbbell in each hand).

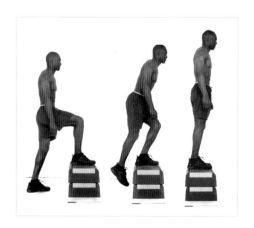

8. Side to side bends + medicine ball

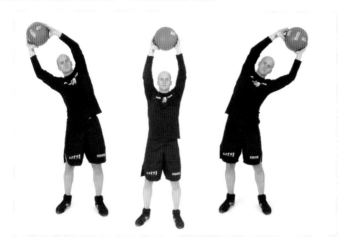

Keep hips square as you slowly bend as far as you can to each side.

9. Side to side seated medicine ball bounce and twist

a) Sit on a mat holding a medicine ball. With knees bent, raise the legs off the floor and bounce the ball from side to side, reaching slightly behind you on each bounce.

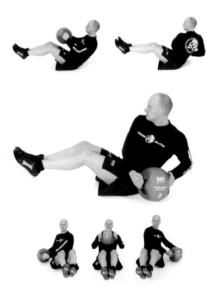

b) Seated side to side medicine ball twist (legs astride)

Sit on a mat with legs astride, turn the medicine ball as far as you can go to each side.

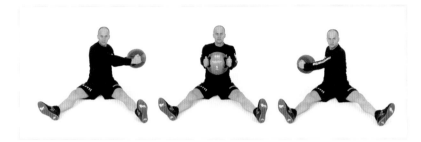

11. Pass-under lunges

Stand with feet shoulder-width apart, holding the dumbbell, medicine ball or a kettlebell in one hand. Lunge forward until both legs describe a right angle then pass the weight under the lead leg into the other hand. Step back and repeat with the other leg.

        a)   with dumbbell

        b)   with medicine ball

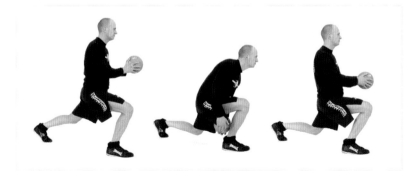

12. Medicine ball pullovers

Lay on your back on a mat with arms extended beyond the head, holding a medicine ball. Sit up to bring the medicine ball over your head while drawing the knees toward the body, and touch the ball down between your ankles. Movement should be continuous.

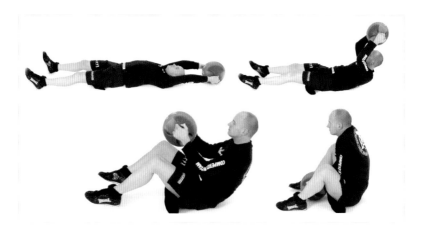

13. Pass-around with medicine ball ('switching')

Sit on a mat with knees bent and legs raised just off the floor. Pass a light (1-2kg) medicine ball behind your back and around to the front. Do this ten times in one direction then reverse the direction for another ten repetitions. As you grow more adept at this exercise, gradually increase the weight.

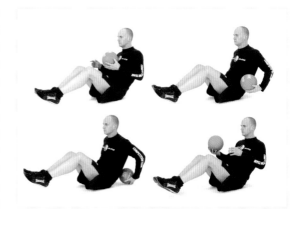

14. Lower abs "tucks" (bringing knees back to chest)

a)   with a medicine ball

Sit on a mat with a medicine ball held between your knees. Lean back 45 degrees, supported by your hands. Raise your legs and draw the medicine ball towards your midriff.

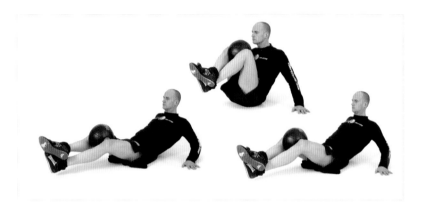

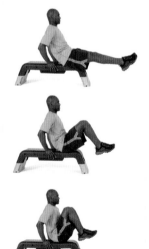

b)   on end of bench

Sit on the end of a bench/step box or similar (as long as it will support you) with your legs extended in front of you. Draw your legs back towards your midriff.

15. Squat thrusts and Burpees

Both are what are now referred to as "old school" exercises, but which are finding a new lease of life as of late.

Squat thrusts; start from squatting position with the hands outside your feet. Thrust your legs out straight behind you until they are fully extended, then return to squatting position.

Burpees: as above, but stand up each time you return to the start position. This makes the exercise slightly harder!

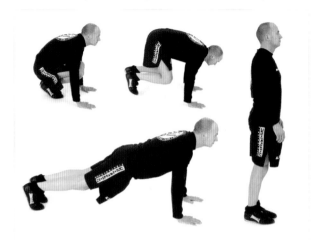

16. Vaults on deck or weights bench

Stand alongside a weights bench, leaning forward and grasping the bench on each side. With feet together, vault the bench from side to side.

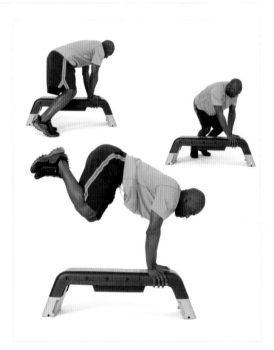

17. Rebounding sit-ups

As with curl-ups, but instead performed facing a wall against which you can bounce a medicine ball each time you come up.

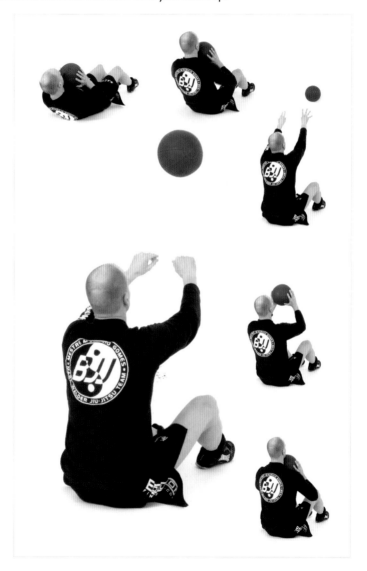

18. Lunge walk with medicine ball twist

Stand with feet shoulder-width apart holding a medicine ball in both hands. Walk forward in alternate lunges, twisting at the waist to turn the medicine ball from side to side with each lunge.

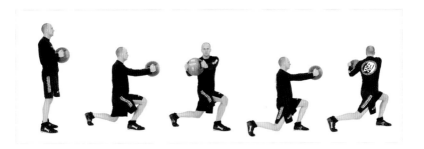

19. Box jumps

Start by standing alongside a step box/ Reebok Deck/ strong crate, then jump sideways, two-footed onto the box, then off the other side to land two-footed.

Graduate to clearing the box as jump two-footed side to side.

Too easy? Try two or more boxes and jump between them, going from side to side.

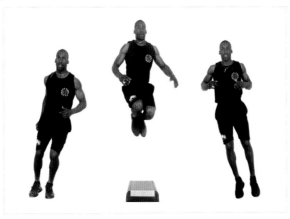

20. Bounding and Hopping

Bounding: place some low hurdles, cones or similar a few feet apart then bound over them to land two footed, spin around and return to start. Start with a one minute set, then progress by half a minute week by week.

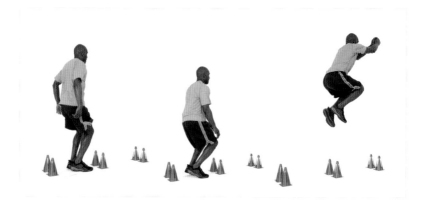

Hopping: as above, but on one leg, changing legs on the return phase.

   a)   forward

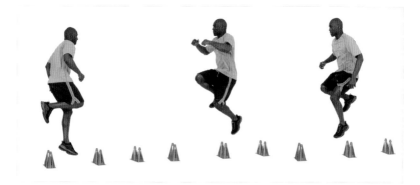

b) sideways

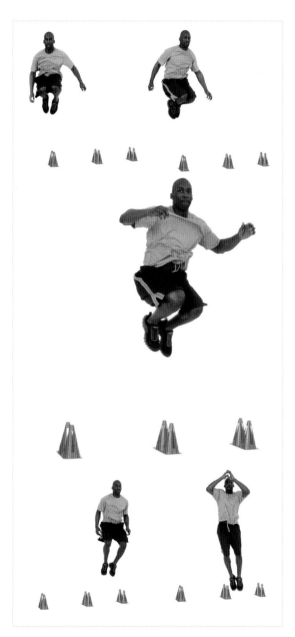

21. Chins

Grasp an overhead bar and pull yourself up to "chin" it. Beat your previous best each with each session.

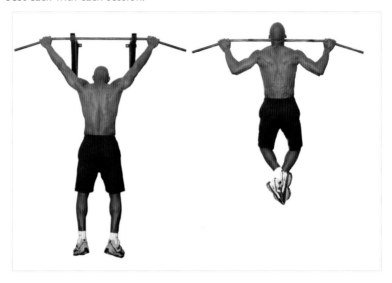

22. Punch bag thrust

Push a heavy bag away from you with a powerful thrust, absorb its return with both hands then repeat.

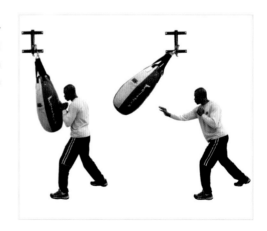

23. Press/push ups

a) Standard press-up

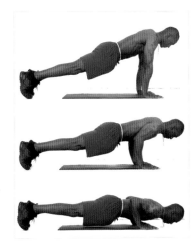

b) Using press-up stands
c) With feet elevated

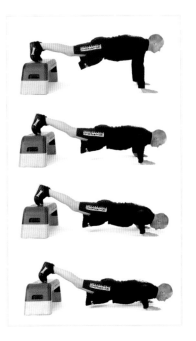

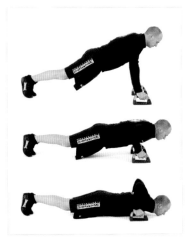

d) With feet elevated using stands

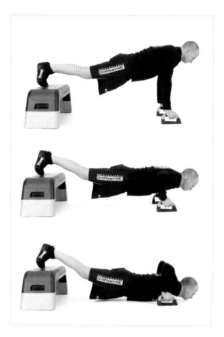

e) With feet on Swiss ball

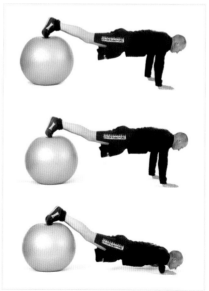

f) With hands on Swiss ball

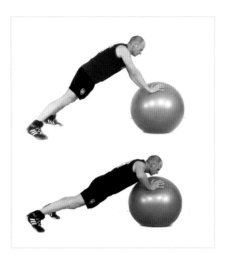

g) With hands on
   medicine ball

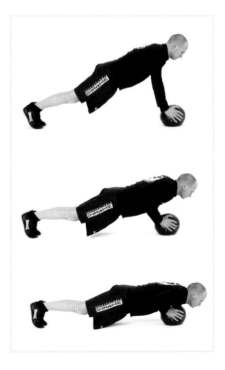

h) With one arm
on medicine ball

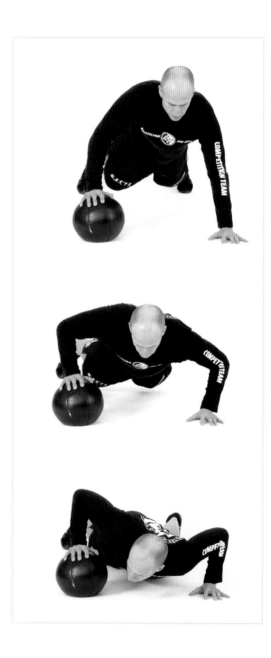

i) Rotational

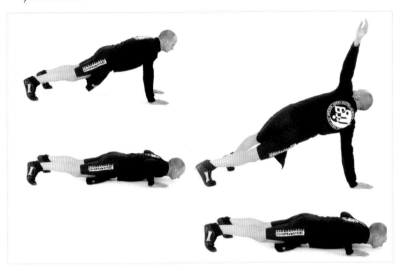

j) Rotational with hexagonal dumbbells

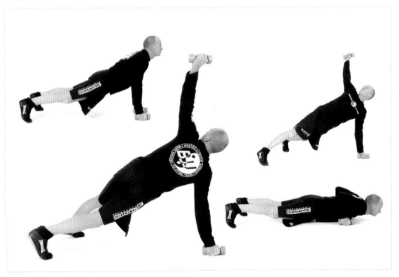

24. Triceps dips on Reebok deck/ bench/strong crate

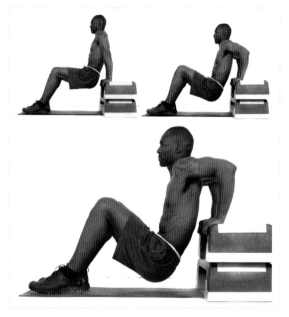

25. Calf raise

Stand on a box with heels hanging over the edge. Go up on your toes and return to drop the heels lower than the edge of the box.

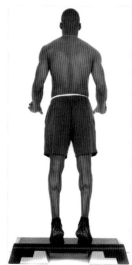

26. Oblique twists, and oblique twists with raised feet

Also called twisting sit-ups. Lay on a mat with knees bent and fingers resting lightly at each side of the head. Raise the trunk, leaving lower back on the floor and twist the upper body so the elbow points at the opposite knee.

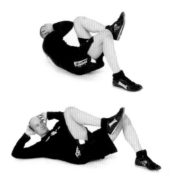

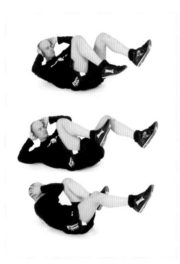

Raising the feet onto a bench makes this a little more challenging.

27. Reverse curls

Lay on a mat with knees bent. Lift your backside off the mat, but not your lower back, taking your knees towards your chest.

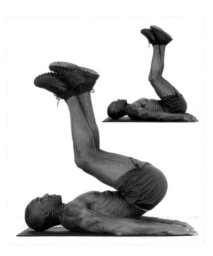

28. Double crunch (knees to elbows)

Lay with your back on a mat with knees bent and fingers resting lightly at the side of the head. Crunch forward and raise the legs simultaneously to meet the elbows.

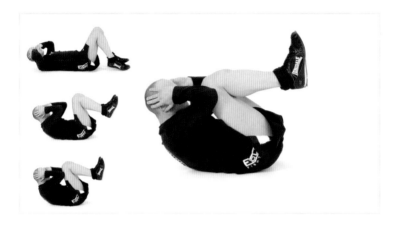

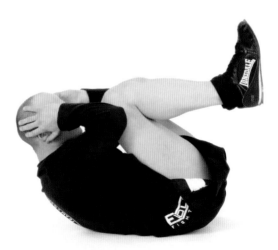

Flexibility and stretching

MAINTAINING FLEXIBILITY, ESPECIALLY AS WE GET OLDER, IS important. It can improve your physical performance as well as your ability to undertake day to day tasks. It should also reduce the risk of injury. Post-exercise stretches will speed your recovery from training, in addition to maintaining or even further developing your level of flexibility.

Thus your training should usually encompass the following phases: the warm-up; the workout; the warm-down; the warm-down stretch.

The warm-up

Cold muscles do not enjoy being stretched. Think of putty or plasticine before you have warmed it in your hands prior to use. If you tried to stretch it in its cold state it would simply tear. Warming-up is essential for three main reasons:

» The body functions better when warm. Warming up enabling the muscles to become more pliable.

» The warm-up helps you focus and prepare mentally for your workout. It, I would hope, puts you in the mood.

» Joint mobilisation. Getting your joints loosened up will get synovial fluid into them. Warming joints up makes this essential fluid runny and more capable of greasing any stiff joints.

Muscles at rest need only 15% of total blood flow, whereas high activity requires 80% of total blood flow as the muscles demand more fuel. The transfer of the supply cannot happen quickly, and so warm-up should be anything from 5–15 minutes, according to the individual and the intended level of exertion.

The activity should be continuous, rhythmic and, ideally, specific or relative to the workout ahead. Always ensure you wear adequate clothing to stay warm;

you can always shed your outer layers when you grow warmer.

To stretch or not to stretch before exercise? The debate rages; the argument revolves around the fact that stretching can leave the muscles in a state that makes exercise more difficult, in complete contradiction to the assumed logic that it makes exercise easier.

For years we were told the importance of a short pre-exercise stretch after warm-up and joint mobilisation, taking 6–10 seconds per body part. The stretch was always performed standing as it was considered that lying down or sitting would allow the body to cool, to the obvious detriment of the warm-up. Suddenly – all change! Fitness gurus seem unable to arrive at a unified agreement on this thorny subject; if you read Christopher M Norris's *The Complete Guide To Stretching* it shows research that stretching reduces 'stiffness' before exercise. However, if you read Jay Blahnik's *Full-Body Flexibility* he claims such stretching could be unhelpful. I consider both books to be splendid guides on stretching and flexibility, but am left none the wiser.

So – what course to take? If you, like myself, have been doing a short stretch (total time of one minute, see end of section) for years and have had no ill-effects or loss of performance, (not that I'd notice much these days) my advice is – carry on regardless.

Why not experiment? Try skipping the short stretch and see if it makes any discernible difference. The sports physiology community changes opinions at such a dazzling pace, I confidently expect it to change in a short time with regard to this subject.

Short stretch after warm-up

(see The One Minute Stretch below, page 151.)

This stretch should be followed by mobility exercises for shoulders, knees, ankles and neck.

Mobilisation

This consist of some simple and reasonably effortless moves to get all the joints limber. Ankles – point the toe and describe small circles clockwise and anti-clockwise.

- Knees – knee bends. Any popping sound effects should die off after the first bend.

- Hips – circle the hips slowly as if exercising with a hula-hoop.

- Shoulders – roll shoulders to and fro, then gently circle the arms to and fro.

- Neck – look over one shoulder, then slowly drop the head forward to scan the floor, lifting the head to look over the other shoulder. Repeat 3-4 times.

Warm-down stretch

One point all fitness professionals will agree upon is that the optimal time for stretching is after your workout, when the muscles are blood-enriched, warm and, therefore pliable. It will help to speed your recovery, reduce muscular soreness and begin the process of waste clearance.

After your workout it is essential to warm down. It also helps to clear lactic acid and reduce muscle soreness; anyone who has ever suffered the dreaded DOMS (Delayed Onset Muscle Soreness) will appreciate the wisdom of avoiding this particular form of agony by a warm-down and a good stretch. This is when you can lay down on your mat and hold those stretches, now that your warm muscles and ligaments are in a receptive state.

The stretches

You can avail yourself of any number of books on flexibility which vary in how much technical information and detailed instruction they provide. I have worked on the basis that for now what you need to know is which muscles to stretch and how to stretch them.

I prefer a system whereby I start at the shoulders and work down, making a return trip to finish off with the neck stretch, which I consider the most important as so many retain stress and tightness here. For this reason I have added extra neck stretches.

You should have warmed up for at least 5 minutes prior to stretching – never stretch cold muscles.

Shoulder stretch

Extend one arm across the chest, then pull it towards you with the other arm.

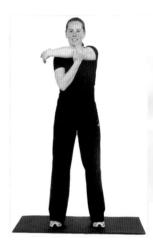

Back stretch (standing)

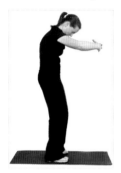

Used in warm-up stretch. With feet shoulder width apart and slightly bent knees, hold the arms out in front, as if clutching a large beach-ball, while contracting abdominal muscles.

Back stretch (prone)

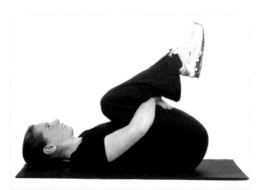

Lying on a mat, pull your bent legs toward you.

Back stretch (angry cat – spinal muscles)

While on all fours, haul in the abdominal muscles while rounding the back like a hump-back bridge.

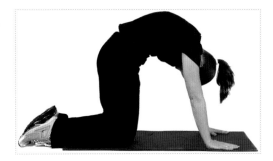

Chest

Hold hands behind your back, raise the arms as you push out the chest.

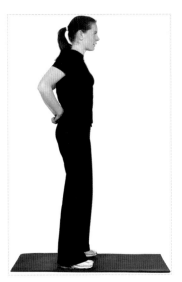

Obliques

Stand with feet shoulder-width apart, raise one arm then list over to the side.

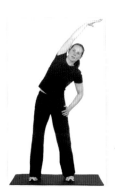

Glutes (the muscles of the backside)

Raise one leg, then place the other leg across it and pull the lower one toward you.

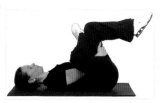

Adductors (muscles on the inside of the legs)

While seated place the soles of the feet to touch each other.

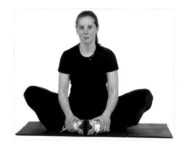

Hamstrings (back of upper leg)

Standing version suited to warm up: raise your leg on a bench or similar surface and keeping upper body straight, lean forward.

Hamstrings

Lying version, suited to warm-down: lay on your back, raise your leg in the air and, holding your calf, pull it towards you.

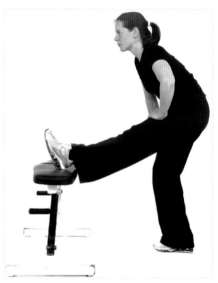

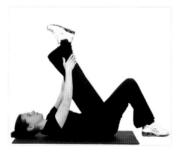

Quads (thighs)

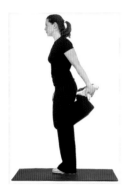

Standing version suited to warm-up: pull lower leg up behind you to touch heel to backside.

Quads

Lying version: lie on front or side, then pull leg back until heel reaches backside.

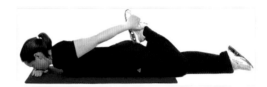

Hip flexors (pelvic area)

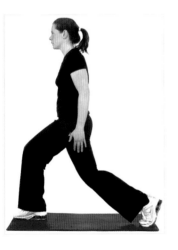

Keep upper body upright as you take a step forward, then lower the hips.

Calf muscles (gastrocnemius, the large calf muscle)

Take a step forward, leaving the heel of the rear foot firmly on the floor as you do. If you cannot feel the stretch, move the rear foot further back until you do.

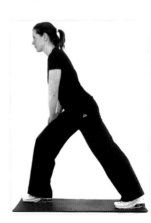

Soleus and Achilles Tendon (lower calf area)

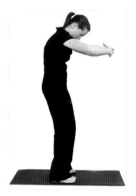

Stand with one foot in front of the other with only a small gap between them. Lower your hips as you bend your knees slightly.

Triceps (back of upper arm)

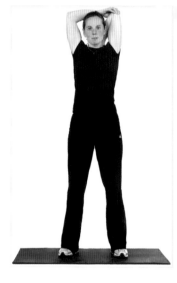

Stand with feet shoulder-width apart and take your arms behind your head. Hold the elbow of one arm and gently pull it behind your head.

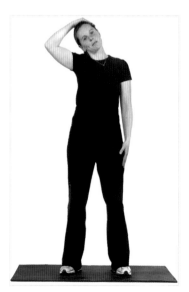

Neck muscles

Place your hand on top of your head, then gently ease the head down toward the shoulder – do not bring the shoulder up to meet it.

Warmed up and ready for the workout? Take a minute for:

The one minute stretch

If you always start at the top and work down there is less chance of missing any muscle group out.

These stretches are held for only 6-8 seconds each. As they usually follow a 5 minute warm-up you are not warm enough to stretch any longer.

Do not hold your breath – breathe naturally.

These are all free-standing stretches, working on the principle you can do them without involving boxes, doorways, mats or any other 'props', so they can be done in a field if necessary.

- *Neck;* look over your shoulder by turning your head slowly to the side. Drop your chin and turn your head to sweep down and across to the opposite shoulder, looking at the ground as you do so. Return to the other shoulder in the same fashion, this will suffice.

- *Shoulders;* raise your left arm straight out in front of you, then, keeping it the same height, take it across your chest until your hand comes in contact with your right shoulder. With your right hand hold the back of the left arm and pull it gently towards the right shoulder. Repeat with the other arm.

- *Back;* with feet shoulder-width apart, bend the knees very slightly. Contract your abdomen while holding your arms out in front of you as if grasping a huge beach ball.

- *Chest;* stand with feet shoulder-width apart with your hands grasped loosely behind your back. Raise your arms behind you and 'lift' your chest as you feel the slight tension applied to it.

- *Hamstrings;* stand with feet fairly close together. Take a large step forward with the left leg. Place the hands flat together against the right (rear) leg. Lift the toe of the left leg until only the heel is on the ground. Keeping the upper body straight lean gently forward, bending the right leg slightly as you do so. Repeat with the other leg.

- *Quads (thigh muscles);* stand with feet slightly apart. Keeping your head up, extend your left arm out to the side, to provide balance as you raise your right leg in front of you. Grasp your instep, and pull it gently up behind you. It may be simpler to just raise your leg behind you and locate your instep as it comes up. Personal flexibility will determine how you achieve it.

  » If you are a little wobbly when trying this, seek out a solid fixture to hang onto with your free hand, (a companion's shoulder will do nicely). Keep the raised leg very close to the supporting leg as you feel the stretch. Repeat with other leg.

- *Calf Muscles;* stand with feet shoulder-width apart, then take a large stride forward with the left leg. Keeping the right leg straight with the heel fully on the ground, bend the left leg and place your hands on the left thigh for support as you bend forward from the waist. Repeat with other leg.

- *Soleus and Achilles Tendon;* stand with one foot slightly in front of the other, where the toe of the rear foot is slightly behind the heel of the front foot. Hands on hips, let your body weight 'sink' down until you feel the stretch at the lower end of the calf muscle of the rear leg. Keep both heels flat on the floor throughout. Repeat with other leg.

Just have a stretch session

The warm-down stretch can be used as a stand-alone session, just so long as your muscles are warm before you start. Consider taking up Yoga, Tai Chi, Pilates or The Alexander Technique if you want to improve your posture as well as your flexibility. A few years ago these disciplines were considered quite alternative, but many martial artists are now using them to improve strength and flexibility, and they are all, in my opinion, worth trying.

It must be considered that weight training will improve your strength, but not your flexibility, which is an equally important aspect of your well-being; so many people have a good weights workout but neglect to stretch properly afterwards.

Flexibility is the best example of a hackneyed, but nevertheless true, maxim: USE IT – OR LOSE IT.

Helpful literature

Sport Stretch Michael J Alter (Human Kinetics)
The Complete Guide to Stretching Christopher Norris (Lyons Press)
Pilates Michael King (Mitchell Beazley)

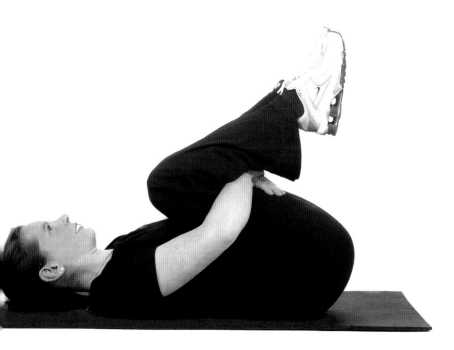

Eating right

IN THIS DAY AND AGE MOST PEOPLE, EVEN schoolchildren, have a pretty accurate idea about the difference between the kinds of foods that are recommended and encouraged, and those that are unhealthy, or even harmful. We are told to get our '5 a day', cut out fatty foods and, in general, make healthy choices. Whether people, armed with this information, will make a healthy choice in the matter is a completely different story. Ironically the unhealthy food, mainly in the form of takeaways and fast food outlets, is chosen because it is regarded as 'cheap' food. In actual fact the cost usually comes not in monetary terms, but in health costs; this stuff can really threaten your state of health, not to mention your waistline.

The good news is that you don't need to starve yourself to lose weight. You are better off eating to lose weight. The secret is to eat the right foods and cut out the wrong ones. There is so much information available with regard to the difference between intelligent eating and downright stupid eating that few can really dispute the fact that they don't know the difference. If you intend to get involved in a serious training programme it really is wise to evaluate what kind of intake you will need to fuel your body for your workouts – and then stick to it. We are unlikely to put fuel into our car that may harm the engine, so why would anybody want to put fuel into their body that they know is potentially harmful?

It is fairly obvious that our diet has a significant influence on our fitness performance. A balanced diet, both in quality and quantity before, after, and in some cases, during activity will greatly benefit performance.

In most cases the balance should be

- Carbohydrate 60-70 %

- Protein approx. 12%

- The remainder will come from fat, which should not exceed 30%

When it comes to dropping a few pounds, a little research into what you should eat is a good start toward a positive outcome. Expert advice on the subject is not hard to obtain. God only knows how many hours of television time are devoted to it.

The good news is that good foods are, in general, more filling, whereas junk food tends to leave you feeling unfulfilled. By improving the quality of your intake you should gradually be satisfied with a smaller volume of food, in which there is a lower percentage of fat, helping you to lower your weight. There is no need, however, to eat food you openly dislike or, worse still, have an allergy to; there is a rich variety of good food available in the shape of fruit, vegetables and starchy food (such as bread, cereal, pasta, potatoes, rice), semi-skimmed milk (skimmed milk always makes me feel as if I'm paying a penance), and lean meats.

If you have the time and the ability (or your partner's ability) try to cook and eat at home, as opposed to getting take-aways or eating out on rich foods. This way you are less likely to add excessive salt or artificial additives of the kind the manufacturers include.

Give your heart a break and cut out unnecessary salt (sodium) from your diet, especially if there is a history of blood pressure or heart disease in your family history. Read food labels and check out the amount of sodium; high levels can be found in salted nuts, crisps and similar snacks, savoury biscuits and hidden in many processed foods such as canned soup, ready-made meals, pickles and sauces and even breakfast cereals. Choose brands with the lowest levels or make your own soups and cereals. Easy guide cookbooks to whip up healthy concoctions that actually taste good have never been more abundant.

When training causes sweat loss to become high it is essential to increase your fluid intake to prevent dehydration. A plastic water bottle to always have by you when training is one of the smartest investments you can make.

Three books, from the many available, I would recommend, mostly because of the writers' credentials but also because they are all relatively inexpensive paperbacks.

Nigel Slater *Real Food* (Fourth Estate)
Rosemary Stanton *Good Food For Men* (Allen and Unwin)
Food For Fitness *Anita Bean* (A & C Black)
Nancy Clark *Sports Nutrition Guidebook* (Human Kinetics)

Food diary

A six month study involving 1,685 middle-aged men and women from four US cities showed that keeping a food diary is a great weight-loss aid. The average weight loss of these individuals was about 13lb; the ones who kept food diaries lost about 18lb, compared to 9lb for those who did not keep a diary. The participants were asked to eat less fat and more vegetables, fruit and whole grains; they were also asked to exercise for three hours a week, mostly by walking, and to attend support meetings.

Dr Victor Stevens, of Kaiser Permante's Center for Health Research in Portland, said "for those who are working on weight loss, just writing down everything you eat is a pretty powerful technique. It helps the participants see where the extra calories are coming from, and then develop more specific plans to deal with those situations."[1]

The study, published in the American Journal of Preventive Medicine, supports earlier research that endorses the value of food diaries in helping dieters lose weight.

Some years ago I encouraged some people I was training to keep a food diary for what I considered a simple reason – anybody who is trying to lose weight will not want to write down "a Mars Bar", "a jam doughnut", "three pints of lager" if they are even semi-serious about losing some weight, as this would be a record of dismal failure.

The record keeping is for your eyes only (I wouldn't have dreamed of asking to see somebody's food diary any more than their personal diary), so you know if you are staying "on the wagon". If the record is not so good at the start and you have to admit to some less than healthy snacks, you will at least have the chance to put the record straight with minor improvements. The secret is to write down absolutely everything you eat and drink.

What I also did was to suggest keeping an exercise diary to run alongside the food diary. It is not rocket science, or even a very exact science, but it will give you some idea of how to roughly calculate how many calories you have taken in and compare it with those you have expended.

Heart rate monitors

Why use a heart rate monitor?

Your heart rate is the most reliable indicator of how hard you are working out, and a heart rate monitor is the best tool yet designed for the layman to employ.

There are more complicated formulae than the basic one that I have chosen – that of subtracting your age from 220 (230 for women). I feel if you are a newcomer to heart monitoring it is the simplest to understand and therefore to use. In time you may want a more advanced system and, if so, my advice would be to obtain a book dedicated to the subject such as *The Heart Rate Monitor Book* by Sally Edwards (Leisure Systems International): just one of several books on Heart Rate Monitors by this author.

Are they expensive?

My Oregon Scientific "Smart Trainer" still costs just under £40, and Polar, the leading and original brand start at around £35 and produce a model specifically for running at around £150.

Getting to grips with it

This health aid was designed by a Finnish professor of electronics, and if you get one, and start getting in too deep, you may wish that you had a similar background in order to set it up. I advocate working on a "need to know" basis; keep it basic for your specific requirements and you should find it can be a terrific help for both fitness and weight management. I somehow resisted the urge to hunt down and flay the fiend who devised the unhelpful Oregon User Manual – it makes getting a pilot's licence seem child's play. The good news is that it does the straightforward job I bought it for – it tells me what my heart rate is when I am training.

Before you can get started you will need to enter your personal data into the monitor. The basic required data is your maximum heart rate.

For this I have used the "Age Predicted Formula", a rough approximation, but cost-free and accurate enough for our purpose. You simply need to deduct your age from 220 (230 for women).

Example
A man of 32 would be 220 - 32 = 188 (Max Heart Rate)
Upper and Lower Limits
You need this to work out your training zone.
For a man of 30;
190 - 30 = 190
190 x 60% = 114 (lower heart rate)
190 x 70% = 133 (upper heart rate)

Training Zones

Heart Rate Intensity	Best for	Best suited to
50% = light	Easy or very long sessions	Beginners
60% = light	Weight management	Everybody (burns up to 85% of calories as fat)
70% moderate	Aerobic training	Fitter individuals improving endurance Moderate length sessions
80% hard	High performance zone	Very fit individuals
90% very hard/ danger zone	Short bursts only	Elite athletes Maintaining superb condition

Your heart rate can drop significantly from the onset of your training as you become progressively fitter, so reassess regularly (I would suggest monthly) and keep a log of your heart rate to keep tabs on your progress,

Important!

Even if you wear a heart rate monitor, continue to be governed by your own instincts regarding your well-being. Never ignore feelings of distress or breathing difficulties – ignore what the monitor is informing you and *stop training*!

The monitor may appear smart and sophisticated but it is only a machine and unable to detect if you are feeling unwell – don't let it dictate to you or become the be-all and end-all of your training.

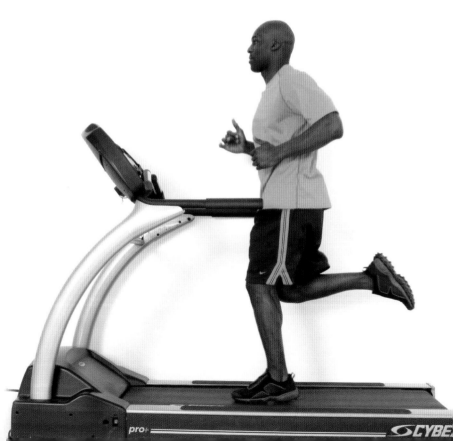

Injury and illness

ONCE YOU START TRAINING YOU CAN GET YOURSELF into great shape, but you also run the slight risk of injury, mild or otherwise.

As soon as you feel any pain or marked discomfort – stop training! Rest the painful area immediately, which will reduce its circulation thereby allowing the tissue to begin the repair process. If you don't know what is causing your pain, describe the symptoms to somebody who you think will know, or who is likely to make a good educated guess and pass you on to the right channels for treatment.

If your injury turns out to be of a long-term nature it does not necessarily mean you cannot train at all. Do what you can, within the bounds of sound sense and comfort. Leg injuries, according to severity, do not mean you can't still train your upper body, just as something like a sprained wrist or elbow ligament problems will not prevent leg training.

Do not put off getting a chronic problem examined professionally. If you get no satisfaction with the National Health Service (some do, some don't, in my experience), consider seeing a private specialist (get an estimate for a single appointment first) – preferably a specialist who has been recommended to you. By doing so you should:

- Find out the root cause of your problem and how to prevent re-occurrence

- Speed up treatment

- Find out how to 'self-help' in the future. If your niggle has been hanging around for a while do some research into it. The web or the public library is almost certain to have something on the subject.

Private treatment is not cheap, but most people will spend more getting their car serviced than getting their leg fixed.

There are books available to teach you how to do your own massage, which is not as tricky as it may at first appear, and which can, with a little patience, prove very beneficial (see "massage and self-massage" below).

Make sure you are warm enough when you train outdoors. Cold muscle fibres do not respond well to being extended. On one of those rare blistering hot summer days, cover your head to protect against sunstroke; train at a cooler time of day.

If you turn up late at the gym don't save time by skipping your warm-up, joint mobilising or stretching – skip an exercise instead.

When buying equipment, as long as you can afford to, go to a store that gives expert advice, be it on weights, footwear, cycles or machines.

When buying any sports shoes, try to do so later in the day when, believe it or not, your feet will be a little larger, by as much as 5%. Tight-fitting shoes can lead to all sorts of foot problems. Blisters are a common problem with people who have recently taken up walking and running for fitness. To prevent them re-occurring, smear the soles of your feet with a coating of Vaseline. Treat blisters by dressing them with a 'blister pack', available from pharmacists, and keep them clean to avoid infection if the skin is broken.

Chronic problems

As stated – if an injury does not show significant improvement with adequate rest and care, or re-occurs when starting training again – seek professional advice.

Illness

There will, inevitably, be times when you will fall prey to the odd cold. The general rule of thumb regarding training is:

* If it's from the neck up (sniffles etc.), train lightly.

* If it's from the neck down (aching limbs, coughing, wheezing, or a feeling of lethargy), do not train at all. Wait for the "all clear" before recommencement.

When returning to training after illness or injury, ease your way back into your regime. You cannot catch up on lost time by overworking, so don't try to.

If friends, family or training partners tell you that you look unwell or off-colour, take notice and proceed carefully; you might just be coming down with something. Curiously enough, nobody wants to share your illness, and gyms are a great place to catch something contagious or infectious, so be considerate.

First aid

Familiarise yourself with the basic procedure to follow if you or a training partner incur an injury. The very minimum you should know and remember is "RICE".

- "R" is for 'rest'. Stop training now!

- "I" is for 'ice'. Get some ice, very cold water or freeze-spray applied to the site of the injury as soon as possible, and try to keep it on for 20 minutes every hour. With ice, wrap in a towel first, to prevent ice burn.

- "C" is for 'compression'. Apply a firm bandage or strapping to prevent painful movement and limit swelling.

- "E" is for 'elevation'. Raise the injured limb to allow blood to flow back to the heart.

This is the most basic explanation of "RICE", but this little information is better than nothing, and quite easy to remember and put into effect. Obviously if the injured person is in apparent agony or has suffered a major trauma, do not do anything other than call for an ambulance as quickly as possible, then make them as comfortable as you can while they wait for professional medical assistance.

A one-day first-aid course is relatively inexpensive and many local councils have them running continuously. Attending such a course counts not only for your own welfare in a crisis, but for friends, family and more usually, total strangers. I signed up for a course many years ago after a youngish man from an opposing football team collapsed with a heart attack in the dressing room, directly after the game and, out of the many people at the ground, only the referee knew what action to take.

Train sensibly

Don't take unnecessary risks like carrying on when in pain, going out running on icy pavements or on foggy evenings.

Never train vigorously in extremes of temperature, especially heat; try to train at the cooler part of the day and ensure you keep your fluid content up.

Try to always get a decent night's sleep, but if you have had a rough, sleepless night don't train too hard the next day.

Achilles tendon and calf problems

The Achilles tendon is a thick strong band stretching from the calf muscle to the heel. The worst injury in this region is a complete or even partial rupture of the Achilles tendon. Not only is it excruciatingly painful, but walking or even standing becomes impossible. A friend who sustained this injury, having been rash enough to jump into a game of five-a-side football with no warm-up, stretching or mobilisation, went down in agony, as if he had been shot. He could not believe he had not been kicked, so sharp and severe had been the pain. The tendon, if completely ruptured, will need to be repaired by being stitched together (sutured) and then immobilised in a cast or splint for six to eight weeks.

Calf pain is a common problem with runners and can occur for a number of reasons, some avoidable, some which need professional investigation to ascertain why they re-occur. The avoidable is usually poor technique or inadequate footwear. Those comfy old trainers may need closer inspection, especially if they have a heel tab that is causing friction, or if the sole is worn and the insole completely knackered out. Go to a specialist running shop for a shoe specific to your needs. If you feel the onset of a nagging pain in the calf while out running/jogging, then slow to a stop and walk to your destination – you cannot 'run it off', it can aggravate the injury considerably. On reaching home, or the changing room, get some ice on it as quickly as you possibly can. After this, carry on the R.I.C.E. procedure and start stretching as soon as the pain subsides, in order to retain flexibility. If walking is difficult try inserting a ready-made heel support of sorbothane or supple sponge rubber.

In addition to the calf stretches shown in the chapter on stretching/flexibility, there are other specific calf stretches you can supplement your recovery with.

The 'Doorstep stretch'

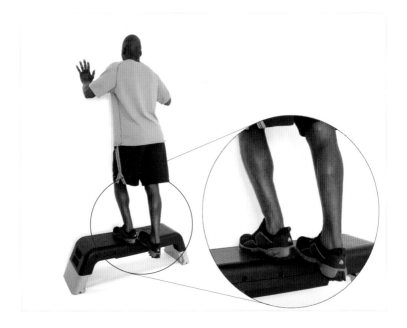

Supporting your upper body, allow your heels to overhang the edge of a step or stair. Lean forward and allow your heels to drop as low as they can. Hold this for 10-15 seconds.

As before but with your heels turned out to give a pigeon-toed effect.

As before but with the heels closer together in a 'ten to two', Charlie Chaplin stance (for more mature readers).

Tiptoe walking

Simply walk around, in bare feet, on the tips of your toes, until your calf muscles ache.

Seated calf stretch

Take an exercise band, towel, or skipping rope and loop it around your bare foot while seated. While pulling on the band, push your toes forward against the resistance. This can be done with a leather or fabric belt if it is long enough to do the job.

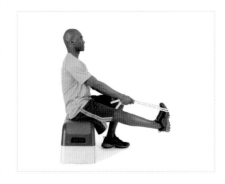

Cramp

Another calf problem is that of cramp; you can, if you are unfortunate enough, get it in various places, but it is usually as you stretch with effort to reach that forehand ground stroke, make that goal-line clearance or similar. You feel a spasm in the back of your lower leg and realise you are, temporarily at least, out of the action. Untrained muscles run the highest risk of falling victim to cramp. The usual course of action, often viewed on weekends at park football matches (professionals only seem to get it in cup finals for some reason) is to lay on the ground while somebody holds your heel and forces the sole and toes of your foot downward. This technique will most likely relieve the spasm, but if it continues a vigorous massage should be tried next. I trained football teams long enough to appreciate the efficacy of both methods, and was thankful of the boring massage course I had once taken. If you have nobody around to manipulate your foot, press your toe against a hard surface, e.g. a wall, a tree and lean forward to stretch the calf muscle. If this fails self-massage comes next. You will need to rub the affected area vigorously, while gritting your teeth in all likelihood.

The causes of cramp are considered to be a deficit of fluid, salt, calcium or magnesium. My personal experience was that habitual cramp sufferers sometimes prevented its onset by eating a packet of crisps an hour or two before a match, purely for the salt content. Others swear by eating a banana or a bowl of cereal and milk; if you are a regular cramp sufferer you can experiment to find your cure, but frequent attacks should be discussed with your G.P. in case there is a serious underlying problem involving blood circulation.

Shin splints

With this injury, pain is felt at the front of the lower leg, along the shinbone. It can often start out as a nagging ache but gradually increase, with activity, into a quite painful and debilitating condition. It is usually caused by landing during running/jogging, football or other activities involving rebounding, on hard or uneven surfaces. Amateur footballers often sustain this injury at the beginning of the season, when their new boots come in contact with hard grounds, as do novice runners setting out on hard pavements. Technique and footwear should both be carefully scrutinised to prevent re-occurrence once recovery is complete and training is resumed.

Self-help involves using ice as soon as possible (see home ice massage kit below). As soon as the pain level allows, start stretching by pulling your toes towards you, preferably against a resistance for more effect. For instance, sit down and insert your toes under a heavy bench, then extend your legs fully until you feel the effect of the action on the injury site. Alternatively get a friend, preferably one of slight build, to stand on your toes as you recline, or press against your feet with their hands.

> Note: both Achilles problems and shin splints can also be caused by increasing the intensity of training too quickly. There is a need to allow time for the body to adapt to increased demands by gradual increments; try not to step up the level of your training too rapidly.

Sprains

Ankle sprain

There are, commonly, two types of ankle sprain, damaging either the lateral (outside area), or the medial (inside area).

a) An inversion injury is likely to injure ligaments on the outside (lateral) side of the ankle. This is the more common injury because there is greater movement in inversion.

b) An eversion injury is likely to injure ligaments on the inside (medial) side of the ankle. This is less common because there is less movement in eversion.

Sprains are generally caused by the ankle 'going over' on an uneven surface, a stumble when moving quickly, or, in my case, missing the edge of a kerb in bad light.

At first you may think, (as I did), "I've only twisted my ankle, it might be all right." When you arrive home the pain has grown, and so has your ankle – usually to twice the normal size.

Your foot starts to feel hot, and the dull ache becomes sickeningly painful and tender to the touch, and any movement is jarring – yes, it's not just a twist, it's a sprain.

Plunge your foot into a bowl, or better still, a 'decorators bucket', a rectangular one, that will allow all the foot to fit in fully extended, fill with cold water and empty the contents of your ice tray into the water – while gritting your teeth, biting on a stout belt etc. Failing this, wrap a packet of frozen peas around the affected side and secure with a tea towel or stuffed down a long sock, and rest your injured leg over the arm of the sofa. From here on follow the R.I.C.E. procedure, but it is always worth getting a doctor to look at the injury, who may suspect a fracture and send you for an X-Ray to make sure.

Once the swelling and pain subside, usually after about one to two weeks, start to exercise your ankle by rotating it in both directions, and with up and down movement of the foot, to improve mobility and flexibility. Roll a tennis ball around with your bare foot to improve strength and control in the ankle.

Wrist Sprain

The wrist is another joint susceptible to sprains, usually incurred by a heavy fall or being wrenched during exercise or working. As before, plunge the affected limb into a bowl or bucket of cold water with a generous helping of ice cubes. As with the ankle it is worth getting a doctor's opinion in case it is not just a sprain but a fracture.

Once the pain and swelling allow, get the joint moving again and try some wrist strengthening exercises using a small dumbbell or a soup can:

Upward roll

Hold the weight over the edge of a bench or table, palm facing upward. Slowly bring the hand up towards you, knuckles facing towards you. Try to do 3 sets of 10 repetitions.

Downward roll

Hold the weight over the edge of the surface with palm facing down. Slowly bring the weight upward as far as you can, with back of the hand facing you. Try to do 3 sets of 10 repetitions.

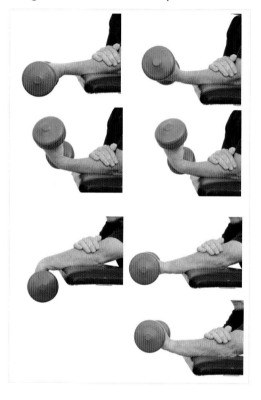

Strengthen the muscles of the forearm by investing in a squash ball or one of those squishy sponge balls made for the purpose (the Gripp lll is a good one) and carry it in the car to use when sitting in traffic, or in your pocket to squeeze while waiting for the bus, tube or train, or while viewing something mind-numbing on television or reading the newspaper – double-tasking that works for everybody.

Massage and Self Massage

Massage is an ancient healing art and can often achieve outstanding results where other healing has failed. It relaxes tired bodies and eases stiff muscles and joints. A session with a professional masseur/masseuse is wonderful, but if you need regular massage it can become expensive. Home massage is an alternative.

In the list of useful literature I have included *Sports and Remedial Massage*, by Mel Cash, (about £15), and *The Complete Guide to Massage* by Susan Mumford, (at about £10). Both have a chapter on self massage, in case you are not in a situation where somebody can give you a massage. The second book is good for total beginners who want to massage or self-massage.

Massage oil can be bought ready-made, but it is equally effective and much cheaper to make your own. Use almond oil or grape seed oil as the carrier oil (the bulk liquid), although baby oil or olive oil will do, and then add the essence of your choice, be it lavender, camomile, peppermint or any from the enormous range available. My personal choice is lavender, not only because a knowledgeable osteopath advised it, but because it smells so good. If you have aching muscles, lemongrass would be a particularly good choice.

The mix: get a plastic bottle that will not leak. You don't want everything in your bag, if you have the oil with you, to reek of essence. Body Shop stores sell empty plastic bottles with a reliable seal for very low cost, as they sensibly recycle all the used bottles customers return. Don't feel tempted to use a washed-out shampoo container; it will almost certainly leak. Fill the bottle up to the shoulders, about 80% full, then add 2-3 drips of essence to a small bottle, the kind you could slip in your washbag, or 7-8 drips into a half-litre bottle. Shake vigorously. A half-litre bottle of grape seed oil from Sainsbury's, Tesco's etc, costs a little over a pound. A bottle of essence from both of the former, or Body Shop, Holland and Barrett or any health store, costs around £3, and lasts for ages. For around £4 you have a long-term supply of massage oil, all you have to do now is rub it in. A massage book will tell you the exact technique, but if you rub towards the heart until the skin reddens, that will be a good start. Apply the oil to warm hands, then to the area requiring massage. Never apply oil directly to the body.

Ice Massage

You can use this handy little device anywhere on the body, but I have found it is extremely useful on strains in the calf muscle.

- Take a Styrofoam cup (one of those that break into thousands of little white balls that get everywhere when crushed), and fill to the brim with cold water.

- Place container in your freezer.

- At the first onset of a mildly strained muscle take the container and cut around the brim with a sharp knife to remove the top half of an inch.

- Massage the hard protruding ice around the injured site until the ice softens and becomes unusable. Concentrate solely on the exact site of the injury – don't widen the area that you ice.

- Time over small areas should be about 5–10 minutes.

- Replace cup in freezer.

- Repeat every time you require it, until it is too small to be practical. For this reason keep two or three on the go at one time. It's a good idea to have two on the go at the same time (a packet of these cups costs under a pound in Tesco).

If the strain is particularly painful use R.I.C.E. procedure instead.

(My sincere thanks to my friend, osteopath Savash Mustafa, for medical advice in this section.)

Helpful reading

Sports Injuries – A Self-help Guide by Vivian Grisogono (John Marshall Books).
First Aid Manual St John's Ambulance (Dorling Kindersley)

It's in the bag – packing for the gym

NOT AS EXTENSIVE AS PACKING FOR A HOLIDAY, but imagine your annoyance when you discover you haven't packed a towel – drying yourself on a sweaty t-shirt isn't quite the same. If you are not the owner of a razor-sharp memory or a born organiser, make a quick list, especially if you are a newcomer to gyms. When buying a sports bag, consider how much kit you intend to tote around; will you be taking your mat/ boxing gloves/handwraps? Some items well worth including, in addition to the obvious showering requirements, are:

- *Flip-flops;* avoid foot infections, particularly verrucas. They are harder to get rid of than a tattoo.

- *Plastic bag;* (a carrier bag will do) to keep your wet stuff away from items you need to keep dry, and avoid getting that "swimming bath" odour in your bag.

- *Water bottle;* stay hydrated, get a large one, fill from the tap and sip as you train. A 'sports' bottle costs around £2-4.

- *Skipping rope;* if you intend to skip at the gym – take your own rope, theirs may all be in use, or too long/short for you.

- *Warm-up gear;* if the gym has a tendency to be on the cool side, i.e. no heating, or somebody has been over-zealous with the air conditioning, throw in a warm sweatshirt, which you can peel off once you are warm. If it is really cold – pack a woolly hat and track trousers. Don't start exercising cold muscles when it is avoidable.

- *Petroleum jelly (Vaseline);* if you are wearing anything new or have some sensitive areas of skin, apply to appropriate areas to prevent chafing and soreness.

- *Small hand towel;* to mop your fevered brow, and any equipment on which you may have left evidence of your efforts.

Also useful

- Small blister pack

- Small packet of plasters

- Small (nail) scissors

- Packet of tissues and medi-wipes

- Safety pins (for emergency clothing repairs)

- Small roll of surgical tape (for repairs to body or kit)

- Pen and small writing pad for note-taking, memos etc.

I feel you are always better off carrying too much than too little equipment.

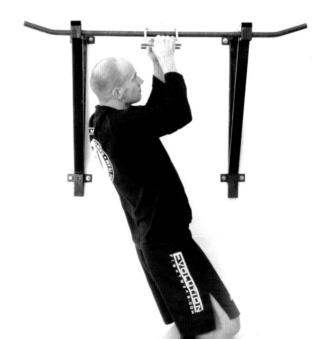

Sample Training Schedules

Cardio Training

I would suggest that beginners start with a rolling sequence of cardiovascular training and weights at a ratio of 2 to 1, as follows:

»   Week 1: cardio two sessions, weights one session

»   Week 2: cardio one session, weights two sessions

»   Week 3: as week 1

»   Week 4: as week 2

Thereafter, as long as you feel fit enough to take on a slightly greater load, progress as follows:

»   Week 5 (and thereafter): cardio two sessions, weights two sessions.

Once this becomes easy, consider yourself at Intermediate level – but this should take months, rather than weeks – don't rush it! Beginners should:

»   Jog/run 20-30 minutes, or

»   Rowing machine 20-30 minutes, or

»   Static Cycle 30-40 minutes, or

»   X-trainer 20-30 minutes

Intermediates should ideally add 10-15 minutes to each of the above, training cardio twice a week.

Advanced should ideally add 20-30 minutes to each of the above, training cardio 2-3 times a week.

Weights Schedules

>> See "Beginners' Charts – machines & free weights"

>> See "Intermediates' Charts – machines & free weights"

>> See "Advanced Charts – machines and free weights"

Full instructions for all exercises quoted here are to be found in the weights chapter.

I have included free weights as I realise not everybody will want to train at the gym. The "free weights" session is equally beneficial (and will save you tapping your foot as you wait for somebody to finish their sixth set on the very machine you are waiting for).

Before every workout

>> Warm-up for 5 minutes with light aerobic work I.e. jogging, skipping cycling etc.

>> Have a 'one minute stretch', page 151.

>> Finish off with a 5 minute cool down (same as warm-up) followed by the 'warm-down' stretches.

Notes for Beginners

Beginners should include 1-2 sessions of abdominal exercises between weights exercises, and progress to abdominal exercises before starting each new exercise (as opposed to resting 30 seconds).

If you are at the gym then all your needs should be catered for. Training at home? You will need the following basic equipment:

a) A set of dumbbells (£15 in Argos at time of writing) which are comprised of one pair of 3kg, one pair of 6kg, one pair of 10kg

b) A bench. On the day of writing I looked on eBay and found a

Weider bench and assorted weights on offer for £28, two York benches for £15 and £16, a ProPower bench for £10 and one by Marcy for £1.20!

c) A mat. A decent Pro Fitness mat at Argos is £3.99. You'll need one of these for a good stretch. If you have a tendency to perspire freely (it's not a crime, in fact in this instance it is to be openly encouraged), give it a generous squirt from an anti-bacterial bottle, such as Dettox. This will prolong its life and prevent it giving off the aroma of mature Stilton.

d) A water bottle. Sip between sets – stay hydrated and you will last longer.

One idea: just before you consign that free local paper to the recycle sack, or use it to line the rabbit's hutch, glance through the second hand weights equipment for sale. Bargains may be found here and, as the aspirations of the more fainthearted fade away, someone else's failure could be the means to your success, as well as the chance to give a decent home to some good quality, but unloved, weights equipment.

New benches at Argos and Tesco Direct start at about £35-40.

Notes for Intermediates

Intermediate Weights Schedule

If training at home, the intermediate trainer will need to add some heavier dumbbells to the list above. Never train at home alone with a heavy barbell; if a dumbbell is too heavy you can put it down again, however quickly and clumsily, but a heavy barbell across the chest can cause injury or, as has happened frequently (I've seen it twice), leave you trapped helplessly on your bench.

As with the beginners' schedule it is not a bad idea to intersperse various abdominal exercises between sets. Perform a single set of abdominal exercises before moving onto your next weights exercise.

Work to a list. Trying to keep it all in your head gets harder as you inevitably tire. Ticking exercises with the aid of a small notebook makes training easier.

Notes for Advanced Training

I would suggest that anybody moving up from Intermediate to Advanced trains at their previous level twice a week and then tries this workout once a week. Once the advanced workout becomes tolerable then switch to using it twice a week, with a couple of days in between. As the advanced workout targets only the chest, back and legs it may be as well to supplement the twice-weekly workout with a light programme involving shoulders, arms and abdominals.

The Advanced Schedules (see charts)

I have given the option of machine or free weights for this workout, as there are only four exercises; you may prefer to mix the equipment up by using the machine for the chest press (advisable if you do not have a spotter) and perform the rest with free weights. The only way you will know what suits you is to experiment, and changing equipment now and again is a sound idea, helping to prevent the workout becoming stale.

I would advise, especially in the first few sessions, to rest 2 minutes between sets, in order to recover from your efforts. The need to lift and lower slowly is paramount.

If you intend to work with a barbell for your bench press (dumbbells are just as good – some experts would say better – as the stronger arm is unable to make the load lighter for the weaker arm when they work bilaterally) make sure your technique is sound:

Grip the barbell, ideally an Olympic barbell, slightly wider than shoulder-width. Ensure your back is flat and your feet are firmly planted flat on the floor. Lower the bar to about an inch above your chest (don't bounce it off your chest), inhaling as you do. Exhale as you slowly drive the bar upward to arm's length. Pause for a second at the top and the bottom of the lift. Take about 3 seconds to complete both the concentric (going up) and the eccentric (coming down) parts of the exercise. Don't forget you need a spotter if you are unsure if you are going to be fully capable of the load. This can eliminate the risk of injury and/or embarrassment.

Important note – do not attempt to lift heavy weights without the aid of a "spotter".

FITNESS TEST GRID

FITNESS TEST	1	2	3	4	5	6	7
1 BLOOD PRESSURE							
2 PULSE							
3 PEAK FLOW							
4 BODY FAT							
5 WEIGHT							
6 WAIST							
7 HIPS							
8 ONE MILE RUN							
9 CHINS							
10 PRESS-UPS							
11 CURL-UPS							
12 PLANK/BRIDGE TIME							
13 BMI							

BEGINNERS' WEIGHT SCHEDULE - MACHINE

Strength Training Log

Start Date:

Exercise		Day 1	Day 2	Day 3	Day 4	Day 5	Day 6	Day 7	Day 8	Day 9	Day 10	Day 11	Day 12	Day 13	Day 14
BENCH PRESS	weight														
	sets														
	repetitions														
LAT PULLDOWNS	weight														
	sets														
	repetitions														
SHOULDER PRESS	weight														
	sets														
	repetitions														
LEG CURLS	weight														
	sets														
	repetitions														
LEG EXTENSIONS	weight														
	sets														
	repetitions														
BICEP CURLS*	weight														
	sets														
	repetitions														
TRICEP PRESSDOWNS	weight														
	sets														
	repetitions														

* BICEP CURLS AND TRICEP PRESSDOWNS ON DEDICATED STATIONS OR ON CABLE STATION

BEGINNERS' WEIGHT SCHEDULE - FREE WEIGHTS

Strength Training Log

Start Date:

BEGINNERS WEIGHTS - DUMBELLS

Exercise		Day 1	Day 2	Day 3	Day 4	Day 5	Day 6	Day 7	Day 8	Day 9	Day 10	Day 11	Day 12	Day 13	Day 14
BENCH PRESS	weight														
SEE PAGE ?	repetitions														
SINGLE ARM ROWS	weight														
SEE PAGE ?	repetitions														
SHOULDER PRESS	weight														
SEE PAGE ?	repetitions														
SQUATS	weight														
SEE PAGE ?	repetitions														
DUMBBELL CURLS	weight														
SEE PAGE ?	repetitions														
TRICEP EXTENSIONS	weight														
SEE PAGE ?	repetitions														

INTERMEDIATES' WEIGHT SCHEDULE – MACHINE

Strength Training Log

Start Date:

INTERMEDIATES' WEIGHT SCHEDULE - MACHINE

Exercise		Day 1	Day 2	Day 3	Day 4	Day 5	Day 6	Day 7	Day 8	Day 9	Day 10	Day 11	Day 12	Day 13	Day 14
FLYES ON PEC-DECK	weight														
	repetitions														
CHEST PRESS	weight														
	repetitions														
LAT PULLDOWNS	weight														
	repetitions														
UPRIGHT ROWS ON CABLE STATION	weight														
	repetitions														
LATERAL RAISE ON CABLE STATION	weight														
	repetitions														
LOW PULLEY BENT OVER RAISE (ON CABLES)	weight														
	repetitions														
LEG PRESS	weight														
	repetitions														
DEADLIFT ON SMITH MACHINE	weight														
	repetitions														
CABLE (BICEP) CURLS	weight														
	repetitions														
TRICEP PRESSDOWNS (ON CABLES)	weight														
	repetitions														

Start Date:

INTERMEDIATE SCHEDULE - FREE WEIGHTS

Exercise		Day 1	Day 2	Day 3	Day 4	Day 5	Day 6	Day 7	Day 8	Day 9	Day 10	Day 11	Day 12	Day 13	Day 14
SKIP	5 MINUTES														
SHORT STRETCH	6/8 SECS														
DUMBBELL FLYES	weight														
	sets														
	reps														
BENCH PRESS	weight														
	sets														
	reps														
SINGLE ARM ROWS	weight														
	sets														
	reps														
UPRIGHT ROWS	weight														
	sets														
	reps														
FRONT RAISE	weight														
	sets														
	reps														
SHOULDER PRESS	weight														
	sets														
	reps														
BENT OVER ROWS	weight														
	sets														
	reps														
SQUATS	weight														
	repetitions														
BICEP CURL	weight														
	repetitions														
TRICEP PRESS	weight														
	repetitions														
DEADLIFT	weight														
	repetitions														
	weight														
	repetitions														
SKIP	5 MINUTES														
WARMDOWN STRETCH															

ADVANCED WEIGHT SCHEDULE

Strength Training Log

Start Date:

Advanced Weights Schedule

Exercise		Session 1	Session 2	Session 3	Session 4	Session 5	Session 6	Session 7	Session 8	Session 9	Session 10	Session 11	Session 12	Session 13	Session 14
5 -10 minute warm up															
Chest press machine on lowest setting or Barbell only	weight														
	repetitions														
	sets														
Bench press (barbell or dumbbells) or Chest press machine	weight														
	repetitions														
	sets														
Single arm rows or 'V' grip pulldowns	weight														
	repetitions														
	sets														
Squats or Leg press machine	weight														
	repetitions														
	sets														
Deadlifts Barbell or Smith machine	weight														
	repetitions														
	sets														
Comments re: difficulty															
5 minute warmdown															

SOLO TRAINING WORKOUT

			1	2	3
	Skip 2 minutes	2 mins			
2	The one-minute stretch	1 min			
3	Shadow box	2 mins			
	Throw jabs, straight rights and hooks from both hands as you move around, remembering the 20 past 12 stance with your footwork. This will get your body heat back up after your stretch and act as a rehearsal for the punch bag. Use only half power in your punching.				
4	Punch bag – on your first session, hit light and fast	2 mins			
5	Skip, at an easy pace	2 mins			
6	Crunches on the floor or Swiss ball	20 reps			
7	Step-ups (10 on each leg) with or without weights	20 reps			
8	Punch bag: solid hitting. Really get stuck in	2 mins			
9	Squats, with or without weights	20 reps			
10	Skip: fast pace	2 mins			
11	Press ups	20 reps			
12	Shuttle run	2 mins			
13	Punch bag (same as #8)	2 mins			
14	Reverse curls	20 reps			
15	Skip: relaxed pace	3 mins			
16	Walk – hands on hips, take deep inhalations to get your breath back	2 mins			
17	Warm down stretch				

Index

Models

My heartfelt thanks go out to all of our models.

Corey Donoghue

Owen Ogbourne

Wayne Rowlands

Steve Wright

Dave Birkett

Victoria Mose

Tanya Rahman